REDISTRIBUTING HEALTH

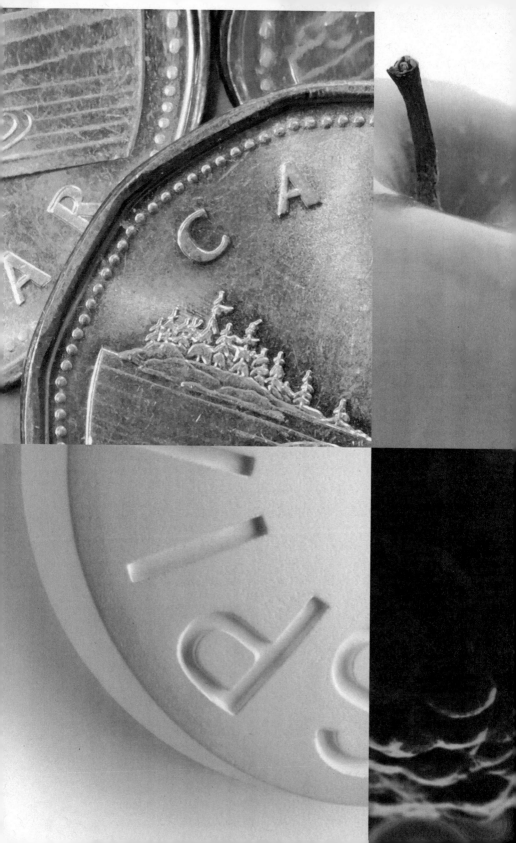

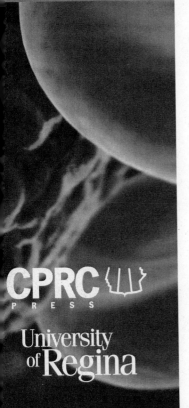

REDISTRIBUTING
HEALTH

New Directions in
Population Health Research
in Canada

edited by Tom McIntosh,
Bonnie Jeffery and
Nazeem Muhajarine

CPRC
PRESS

University
of Regina

with a foreword by André Picard

Printed and bound in Canada at Friesens.
The text of this book is printed on 100% post-consumer recycled paper.

Cover and text design: Duncan Campbell, CPRC.
Infographics on pages 82, 85, 141, 143 and 145 by Duncan Campbell, CPRC.
Editor for the Press: Donna Grant, CPRC.
Index by Patricia Furdek, Ottawa, Ontario.

COVER PHOTOS: "Single aspirin pill, close-up," Ocean Photography/Veer; "Granny Smith Apple," Corbis Photography/Veer; "Canadian Dollar Coins," © Sam Shapiro/Fotolia.com; and "Blutzellen und Krebszelle," © Sebastian Kaulitzki/Fotolia.com.

Library and Archives Canada Cataloguing in Publication

Redistributing health : new directions in population health research in Canada / edited by Tom McIntosh, Bonnie Jeffery and Nazeem Muhajarine ; with a foreword by André Picard.

(Canadian Plains proceedings, 0317-6401 ; 38)
Papers presented at a conference held in Regina, Sask., in November 2008.
Includes bibliographical references and index.
ISBN 978-0-88977-227-4

1. Health—Social aspects—Canada. 2. Health—Social aspects—Research—Canada. 3. Equality—Health aspects—Canada. 4. Equality—Health aspects—Research—Canada. 5. Public health—Social aspects—Canada. 6. Public health—Social aspects—Research—Canada. I. McIntosh, Thomas A. (Thomas Allan), 1964- II. Muhajarine, Nazeem, 1962- III. Jeffery, Bonnie, 1953- IV. Series: Canadian plains proceedings 38

RA440.87.C3R44 2010   362.1'0420971   C2010-905262-5

10   9   8   7   6   5   4   3   2   1

CPRC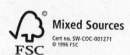
PRESS

Canadian Plains Research Center
University of Regina
Regina, Saskatchewan, Canada, S4S 0A2
TEL: (306) 585-4758   FAX: (306) 585-4699
E-MAIL: canadian.plains@uregina.ca   WEB: www.cprcpress.ca

We acknowledge the financial support of the Government of Canada through the Canada Book Fund for our publishing activities, the support of the Canada Council for the Arts for our publishing program.

 Canadian Heritage   Patrimoine canadien   Canada Council for the Arts   Conseil des Arts du Canada

Mixed Sources
Cert no. SW-COC-001271
© 1996 FSC
FSC

Contents

Foreword—*André Picard*

vii

Introduction: Moving Forward on Critical Population Health Research
— *Tom McIntosh, Bonnie Jeffery, and Nazeem Muhajarine*

xi

SECTION 1: THEORY AND ETHICS

The Essential Value(s) of Health: Implications for Canadian
Population Health Research and Policy—*J. David Guerrero*

3

Towards an Ethical Framework for Population Health
Research in Canada: A Place for Ethical Space?
—*Sylvia Abonyi, Shanthi Johnson, Diane Martz, Tom McIntosh,
Nazeem Muhajarine, and Bonnie Jeffery*

20

Income Inequality and Health:
A Theoretical Quagmire—*Nadine Nowatzki*

35

SECTION 2: CRITICAL POPULATION HEALTH

Aboriginal Health Research and Epidemiology:
Differences between Indigenous and Western Knowledge
—*Ulrich Teucher*

57

The Shifting Discourse of "Public Participation": Implications
in Changing Models of Health System Regionalization
—*Kelly Chessie*

74

"A Healthy Pregnancy is in Your Hands": Agency, Regulation,
and the Importance of Social Difference to Women's Experiences
of the Medicalization of Pregnancy—*Janelle Hippe*

93

SECTION 3: POPULATION HEALTH IN PRACTICE

Dragon Boat Racing as an Alternative Type of
Support for Women Living with Breast Cancer
—*Rhona Shaw*
115

Integrating Population Health Promotion and Prevention:
A Model Approach to Research and Action for Vulnerable
Pregnant Women—*Angela Bowen and Nazeem Muhajarine*
133

The Cousin of Globalization:
Neo-liberalism and Child-Relevant Policy
—*Jennifer Cushon and Nazeem Muhajarine*
151

List of Contributors—**171**

Index—**173**

Foreword

André Picard

Eat your veggies, exercise, keep your weight down, and don't smoke: It's an appealing formula for good health and longevity, and one that predominates in the public consciousness.

If only it were so simple. Lifestyle plays a role in the health of individuals, and so does genetics. But social justice—or lack thereof—has a greater impact on the health of the population than the human genome, lifestyle choices, and medical treatment.

It is virtually impossible to fathom that a person could truly be healthy without some basics: a roof over one's head, decent food on the table, an adequate income, an education, a modicum of control over one's daily life, and a secure place in the community. Only then can we have the luxury of wondering if we have sufficient omega-3 fatty acids in our diet and puzzling over the relative health merits of yoga versus tennis.

These statements should come as no surprise to readers with an interest in population health issues; if anything, they will be seen as self-evident. The scientific evidence demonstrating the importance of socio-economic determinants to the health of individuals and, more importantly, to the health of populations, is overwhelming. And, as demonstrated by the essays in this book, our understanding of these concepts is increasingly sophisticated.

However, the discussion surrounding population health, unfortunately, remains largely the purview of academics and occurs in the confines of conferences like "New Directions in Population Health Research: Linking Theory, Ethics, and Practice." These concepts, and the discussion of how we can apply our knowledge of socio-economic determinants of health and population health to actually improve the health of the population, need a broader audience. Put another way, in addition to making links between theory, ethics, and practice, there is a need to reach a broader audience, well beyond those who have an obvious stake in this research.

For population health research to have a real impact, the larger public needs to be engaged. The real challenge in the field of population health is not to map precisely the correlation between income and health outcomes; it is to get the basic discussion of the importance of that link on the public policy radar.

Currently, we pour vast amounts of money into treatment, dealing with the proximate causes of disease, but we have virtually ignored prevention, particularly the most effective prevention of all, creating social conditions that foster good health. This approach to medicine and health is much like closing the barn door after the horse has escaped: It fails to address what Sir Michael Marmot calls the "causes of the causes of poor health." There is little point in trying to prevent and treat illness in the absence of social justice, and there is a pressing need to tackle the root causes of injustice, including poverty, poor housing, gender inequality, inadequate education, and lack of respect for human rights.

So why do we fail to do so?

Health is an intensely personal issue. Yet, the factors that have the greatest impact on health, both on an individual and population level, are societal. That's scary. As an individual, I want to believe that I have control over my health; when you start telling me that because I have a low-paying job I have a higher risk of heart disease or depression, it leaves me feeling impotent.

Health is also reactive, and deeply emotional. In everyday life, healthy people don't worry that much about health issues—unless they're women, and then they worry about the health of their children and their parents, not about their own health. Then, when health *is* an issue, they quickly lose sight of the big picture. When they are sick with colon cancer, or a family member is beginning to suffer from dementia, they want answers, they want practical information, and they want care. They don't want to hear about the need for a minimum wage that ensures a decent income, about the lack of social housing, and about gender inequality.

The structure of our health and social welfare system has greatly facilitated this short-sightedness. Many of us revel in thinking of Canada as a great place to live—a generous, caring country with a well-woven social safety net that protects the sick and poor from harm. However, that "feel good" image is largely a myth.

While we have a generous health care system—our beloved medicare— Canada's welfare system is parsimonious at best. The examples are many:

- minimum wage (which varies by province) is inadequate, to the point where one-third of full-time workers cannot make ends meet;
- only about one-third of people who are unemployed are actually eligible for employment insurance;
- almost 40 percent of all jobs are part-time or seasonal;
- there are 1.2 million poor children in Canada, and nearly 320,000 of them rely on food banks for their daily bread;
- welfare rates (which vary by province) provide income well below the poverty line;
- our social programs have perverse disincentives, such as those that require people to quit their jobs and go on welfare to get catastrophic drug coverage;
- there is shocking poverty among native peoples; not surprisingly, their health is abysmal;
- child care is inadequate almost everywhere;
- there is an army of unpaid caregivers who have virtually no official help;
- social housing is virtually non-existent.

In Canada, only 17.8 percent of public expenditures are on social programs other than health; in Sweden, by contrast, that figure is 36.8 percent. According to the Organization for Economic Co-operation and Development, 21 European countries spend more on social programs than Canada does, including Poland and the Slovak Republic. Not coincidentally, all of those countries also spend less than Canada on health.

The countries that are healthiest are not necessarily the wealthiest. Rather, they are those where disparities between the richest and poorest are the smallest. The lesson we should be taking from European countries is that one of the most effective health interventions is income redistribution. To ensure good population health, we need to invest in a social safety net.

In modern society, we place an inordinate amount of attention on how we live and on our lifestyle, but not nearly enough on how those around us live. We focus too much on controlling disease with prescription drugs, surgery, and other interventions, but not nearly enough on ensuring our physical, mental, and social well-being.

Money is the best drug we have. And, paradoxically, providing people with a decent income is probably cheaper than treating the illnesses of poverty, which tend to be expensive conditions such as diabetes, heart disease, and cancer. Yet welfare—quick shorthand for social programs that redistribute wealth—has become a dirty word, particularly in political circles. We love our health care system (which is more accurately described as a sickness care system) and, increasingly, we hate welfare. Yet it is a false dichotomy and a false economy. We can pay now with decent social programs or pay later with increased health costs.

So, how do we bridge that gap? How do we get the general public to grasp and embrace the notion that investing in population health will ultimately result in better personal health?

There is no easy answer to that question. But, there are certainly some lessons to be learned from other areas of the health care sector. The groups that have had the greatest influence on public policy in recent years are those in the chronic disease field, the ones the media refers to as the "disease-of-the-week" gang: arthritis, Alzheimer's, autism, colitis, breast cancer, heart disease, etc. What these groups have done is to take sprawling issues and make them compelling to the general public by putting a personal face on them. Disease groups—in highlighting personal tales of tragedy and triumph—have also, paradoxically, helped create a collective sense of responsibility among the public. We all have a personal stake in cancer—or at least we feel we do.

The challenge facing the field of population health is precisely that one: To make the public feel a collective sense of responsibility for social imbalances and injustices and a desire to conquer them.

Imagine for a moment the impact on our collective health and well-being if we were as committed to conquering poverty as we are committed to conquering cancer. The much-ballyhooed war on cancer has more than its fair share of basic scientists, academics, and clinicians on the front lines, many with contradictory theories and practices; it has its epistemological, ethical, and scientific disagreements; it has its successes and failures. But, most important of all, the research findings, clinical practice changes, and ethical challenges do not occur in a void. They matter to the general public.

Population health research will have a meaningful impact only when population health is part of the public discourse, not dismissed as a marginal element in social, economic, and political debate.

INTRODUCTION
Moving Forward on Critical Population Health Research

Tom McIntosh, Bonnie Jeffery, and Nazeem Muhajarine

INTRODUCTION

The papers collected in this volume stem originally from a conference, "New Directions in Population Health Research: Linking Theory, Ethics, and Practice," held in Regina, Saskatchewan, in November 2008. The conference was sponsored by the Saskatchewan Population Health and Evaluation Research Unit (SPHERU)—an interdisciplinary research unit composed of faculty from both the University of Saskatchewan and the University of Regina—and the Community and Population Health Research (CPHR) training program—a strategic training initiative funded by the Canadian Institutes of Health Research (CIHR) and administered by SPHERU faculty that offered research, training, and mentorship to an interdisciplinary mix of graduate students, post-doctoral fellows, and community-based researchers.

The "New Directions" conference held over 40 panel presentations, 16 poster presentations, and a number of plenary sessions over two and a half days. The over 200 registrants and presenters came from all parts of Canada and abroad. They shared not only an overarching commitment to the general furtherance of population health research, but also a commitment to a particular conception of that research—one that is theoretically and epistemologically sophisticated, strongly empirical (both quantitatively and qualitatively), meaningfully engaged with the populations it purports to speak about, critically self-aware of the ethical challenges and power dynamics of collaboration with populations who may be marginalized and excluded in various ways, and aimed at change—in policy, in politics, in outcomes, and in the socio-economic dynamics that underpin the health of those populations. It is this approach to critical population health research that is at the heart of SPHERU's mission and that of the CPHR training program, which sought to train, mentor, and support the next generation of population health scholars, researchers, and community builders.

The following pages provide an overview of SPHERU, the CPHR training program, and the volume itself. The goal is to present an understanding of how SPHERU sees itself and its mission both as a research unit and, through the CPHR training program, as a teaching unit. That exploration provides not only the rationale for the volume, but also an understanding of how the volume is a logical outgrowth of SPHERU's mission and a reflection of SPHERU's and CPHR's places within a larger research community and project.

We begin by revisiting two quite different but complementary statements of SPHERU's contribution to a larger research and political project called "critical population health." From here, a more focused look at the elements of SPHERU's current research agenda helps situate the unit within the universe of critical population health research in the country. Discussion of the CPHR training program adds another important dimension as it emphasizes the role SPHERU plays in creating an interdisciplinary environment where a new generation of critical population health scholars emerges. Finally, a small selection of studies, presented at the "New Directions" conference, illustrate the diverse approaches and emphases of critical population health research.

Critical Population Health: Research and Project

In 2005, SPHERU faculty articulated an understanding of the essence of their "*critical* population health research project." That project was defined as having two interrelated goals:

> (1) a thoroughgoing deconstruction of how historically specific social structures, economic relationships and ideological assumptions serve to create and reinforce conditions that perpetuate and legitimize conditions that undermine the health of specific populations; and (2) a normative political project that, as a result of deeper understanding, seeks the reconstruction of social, economic and political relations along emancipatory lines. (Labonte et al., 2005, p. 6)

The first goal speaks to the "research" element, a deep understanding of how social, economic, and political structures came to be and how they came to be seen as legitimate in spite of the fact that they unequally distribute health amongst populations. This lies at the heart of a critical approach to understanding the determinants of population health. The second goal speaks to the idea of critical population health research as a "project." The deconstruction of how specific determinants of health operate in specific historical and contemporary contexts is ultimately of little, other than academic, interest (both literally and figuratively) if it is not undertaken as part of a conscious agenda to bring about social, political, and economic change in those contexts. The end result(s) of both the "research" and the "project" has to be the increasingly equitable distribution of health creating and sustaining conditions within and between populations.

The "research" and the "project" become interrelated and the distinction between them blurs through the active and sustained engagement of the researcher with theory, community, and policy. The multidisciplinary nature of population health research requires researchers to be explicit about the epistemological assumptions that they bring to their work from their respective disciplines. It is through this continued assessment and critique of those epistemological stances that critical population health research attempts, though with varying degrees of success, to move itself from being merely multidisciplinary to being inter- or transdisciplinary in its undertakings. And that critical self-reflexivity becomes important in research that attempts to understand the cultural specificities of those populations within a society for whom traditional Western epistemologies have no resonance or purchase. This has been a key challenge for SPHERU in its engagement with Indigenous communities. "The most ambitious resolution to these questions, to date, has been adopting the principle of 'ethical space', where different world-views are exchanged and discussed until some shared statements arise about the nature of research, questioning, analysis, and dissemination are reached" (Labonte et al., 2005, p. 11).

The ongoing engagement with policy (and with policy-makers) remains a particular challenge for critical population health researchers because of the political nature of the research project itself. Policy change is almost always incremental and takes place within a context that rejects any wholesale repudiation of the ideological constructs of the dominant social and economic order. Thus, the population health researcher who approaches "policy relevance" with a presumption that necessitates the wholesale reconstruction of social, political, and economic institutions is almost certain to fail to seriously engage the preternaturally conservative policy processes of contemporary liberal-democratic capitalist states. But policy windows do open when problems, solutions, and politics align around certain issues (Kingdon [1995] 2003, 2006), and researchers who can effectively engage in a dialogue with policy-makers can effect some beneficial changes to health-determining conditions or ensure some measurable increase in their more equitable distribution.

Writing in *The Lancet* in 2008, SPHERU again articulated a research agenda centred on a direct engagement with both communities and policy-makers around the determinants of health that at once held true to the "emancipatory" goal of a critical population health research project while understanding the likelihood of policy change as incremental (Johnson et al., 2008, pp. 1690–1693). Building on governments' own commitments around the determinants of health, SPHERU noted that a national population health framework for Canada that

> is responsive to evolving knowledge on social determinants of health, and which integrates considerations for structure, process, and funding, holds promise for achievement of goals for reduction of health disparities. The national framework needs to explicitly include linkages with jurisdictions, sectors, and stakeholders. Short-term and long-term goals, objectives, and targets are important for the framework to have the greatest chance of influence in the reduction of health disparities. (p. 1690)

It is the oft-times incomplete nature of policy change that continues to drive the necessity for re-articulating the emancipatory project inherent in critical population health research. However frustratingly slow the incremental change is, it is important to keep in mind that inequitable distribution of health and health-sustaining conditions is not an abstract, theoretical construct. It is about real people and real communities facing real challenges, and it is also about the fact that those challenges are transmitted across generations. Lessening those challenges, increasing the health of those communities, and improving the likelihood that subsequent generations will be healthier than past generations is, ultimately, emancipatory.

SPHERU's Mission

SPHERU's mission *to promote health equity by understanding and addressing population health disparities through policy-relevant research* is addressed by actively involving communities, community organizations, non-governmental organizations, and policy- and decision-makers in both the research enterprise itself and in the communication and application of research results. SPHERU researchers are committed to the belief that this more open and collaborative research approach allows us to accomplish the unit's overall goals, which are to:

1) mobilize and build on the existing expertise of a diverse group of researchers, trainees, and students acting collaboratively;

2) mobilize and build on the existing knowledge and capacity (for research and uptake) of our research partners;

3) ensure that the research questions we ask and the results our research generates speak directly to improving the health of Saskatchewan residents; and

4) make the exchange of research knowledge with communities and policy-makers more seamless through this ongoing engagement with each other, our partners and the broader research and policy communities.

The thematic focus of critical population health research should be shaped by a consideration of the interests of those who face the greatest burden of disease. Thus, reflecting our group's interdisciplinary expertise, SPHERU faculty apply a critical population health approach in three areas of focus that represent a significant proportion of vulnerable peoples in intersecting contexts of vulnerability. While the description presents a discussion around each research theme area independently, there is significant overlap among them, both in reality and from a population health perspective.

Our research themes—healthy children, northern and Aboriginal health, and rural health—derive directly from our understanding that the health status and health outcomes of these populations and in these settings are particularly relevant to Saskatchewan. Our focus on these specific areas along with our attention to building our research in collaboration with communities and policy-makers and our attention to the most effective ways of translating and disseminating our research findings have been identified as priority health research areas for Saskatchewan (Saskatchewan Health, 2004; Sinclair, Smith, & Stevenson, 2006). While SPHERU is committed to engaging in theme-focused research of particular relevance to Saskatchewan, it must be noted that knowledge produced in these thematic areas will have an impact on jurisdictions both closer to and farther removed from Saskatchewan. How societies respond to their children, their cultural and language minority populations, and their communities (which are increasingly "distanced," not just geographically but also in influence) are currently issues of great importance in Saskatchewan and elsewhere.

Healthy Children

Children are an example of a population group where compromised health has consequences, not only for their life course, but also for society. SPHERU's research in this area addresses the limitations of previous studies and incorporates a critical population health approach.

Overall, work in the area of healthy children contributes, first, to a deeper understanding of how the various contexts (family milieu, neighbourhood social and physical environment, and school environment) shape child health and developmental outcomes and, second, to learning how successful our community-based intervention efforts are in producing better outcomes for children. Through this research and by working closely with decision-makers, SPHERU contributes to achieving better health and development for all children in Saskatchewan.

Northern and Aboriginal Health

SPHERU's research in the area of northern and Aboriginal health is situated in the global context of Indigenous frameworks and indicators discourse, and broadly framed through the lens of culture as a health determinant. We know that peoples around the world continue to experience disproportionate health burdens, with large disparities in most social and health indicators (Bramley et al., 2005; Jebamani, Burchill, & Martens, 2005).

Bramley et al. (2005, p. 849) observe that "to measure progress toward reductions in health disparities, it is essential that quality Indigenous health data exist." This requires conceptual level progress in the area of culturally relevant definitions of health, accompanied by the development of indicators suitable to these new frameworks (Jeffery, Abonyi, Labonte, & Duncan, 2006). Both of these areas of research are unfolding in a national and global context that explicitly recognizes culture as a health determinant (Smylie & Anderson, 2006) but is constrained in its application (Wilson & Rosenberg, 2002) by our weakly developed understanding of what that means (Dressler & Bindon, 2000) and how culture intersects with other, better-defined determinants such as income, social status, education, and employment (Dressler, Oths, & Gravlee, 2005). SPHERU's projects explore the role of culture in population health by looking at culture as a *determinant* of health, by considering culturally relevant *definitions* of health, and through refining cultural identity as an *indicator* of health.

Rural Health

Rurality is a powerful determinant of women's and men's health. "How Healthy are Rural Canadians?" (DesMeules & Pong, 2006) illustrates their poorer health status, points to significant inequities in health-determining conditions compared to their urban counterparts, and identifies some of the contextual factors unique to rural settings that may exacerbate or mitigate health outcomes of rural residents.

Saskatchewan is one of the most rural provinces in Canada, with at least 36 percent of its population living in rural areas (Romanow, 2002) that have been hard hit by economic restructuring in agriculture and forestry, the loss of young people, deteriorating infrastructure, and the restructuring of the provision of services in health and education (Martz & Sanderson, 2006). The economic crises in the resource sectors have increased the impact of poverty in rural regions, necessitating a better understanding of the inter-relationships between rural poverty and the health of rural women and men. Economic and social change has also led to changing roles and relationships for both women and men in rural communities, some of which challenge traditional rural cultures (Martz et al., 2006).

Studies of healthy lifestyles and risk behaviours that focus on rural youth are rare, and most studies of youth risk behaviours in Canada make no distinction between rural and urban youth. In this context, understanding the role of rural culture as an influence on healthy lifestyles and risk behaviours among rural youth will provide a much stronger basis for program planning for Saskatchewan rural youth. Rural health research projects conducted by SPHERU will provide a better understanding of the impact of social and economic determinants on the health of rural women, men, and youth through the application of a population health approach. Our goal is to provide grounded, comparative, and comprehensive analysis of the impact of social and economic change on the health of women, men, and youth living in rural Saskatchewan. SPHERU's research actively involves people living in rural communities, as well as policy-makers and practitioners who design and implement health policy in Saskatchewan in order to inform strategic and policy options.

Knowledge Mobilization, Transfer, and Exchange

SPHERU's research is linked to sophisticated and multi-faceted strategies of knowledge mobilization, transfer, and exchange with fellow researchers, policy-makers, and communities. These strategies are operationalized depending on the nature of the research and, in the case of collaboratively driven research, are part of the research strategy from its conception. These knowledge mobilization, transfer, and exchange activities are the vehicles through which the research team helps to build the capacity of researchers, students, policy-makers, and communities to take action to address the determinants of health in a manner that can reduce health inequities.

TRAINING THE NEXT GENERATION OF (CRITICAL) POPULATION HEALTH RESEARCHERS

SPHERU's efforts in population health do not end with the practice of its particular brand of research but extend to training the next generation of researchers who will sustain and advance a critical population health research agenda. This "teaching and training" mandate, primarily promulgated by the innovative CPHR training program, has coalesced around SPHERU. The program itself is larger in scope since it draws expertise from multiple disciplines at the University of Saskatchewan and the University of Regina.

The CPHR training program, like other strategic training programs in health research in Canada, is timely, has attracted high-performing trainees, and creates an interdisciplinary milieu of junior and senior scholars who thrive in the scholarly interchange of give and take. The training program is built on three key elements: a transdisciplinary training environment bridging two universities of higher learning, the belief that knowledge translation and exchange are essential components of advanced research competency, and a commitment to strong mentorship that 'glues' the program together.

The first of these elements, *transdisciplinary research and scholarship,* is much in vogue in academic circles but is often loosely defined and is used synonymously with related terms such as multidisciplinary or interdisciplinary research. As Nicolescu (2008) asserts, transdisciplinarity concerns a perspective, engagement, and action that is at once between the disciplines, across the different disciplines, and beyond each individual discipline. Its goal is the understanding of the present world from different perspectives (or realities), of which one of the imperatives is the overarching unity of knowledge through integration. Transdisciplinarity as a principle of integrative forms of research comprises a family of methods for relating scientific knowledge, lived experience, and the practice of problem-solving. In this understanding, transdisciplinary research addresses real world issues, not just abstract ideas. Transdisciplinarity asks whether and to what extent an integration of different scientific perspectives is addressed. This aspect is often used to distinguish between trans-, inter-, and multidisciplinarity. While not a new discipline or a superdiscipline in itself, transdisciplinarity often creates new understandings and is nourished by disciplinary research; in turn, disciplinary research is clarified by transdisciplinary knowledge in a new, fertile way.

This transdisciplinary perspective is a perfect complement to population health research and scholarship, since the field of population health itself is an integrative science—rather than a discipline—and is fundamentally concerned about health problems in the real world. In SPHERU—CPHR we have assembled scholars and scholars-in-training who are schooled in specific disciplinary, epistemological, and methodological perspectives, but have entered a space that allows learning, understanding, and working across disciplines. Understanding this transdisciplinary research can only arise if the participating actors interact in an open discussion and dialogue, accepting each perspective as equally important, and relating the different perspectives to each other. We have created opportunities and mechanisms for CPHR trainees and mentors to allow this interchange to occur. The program is designed to create spaces for transciplinarity to take root, including an introductory retreat, a closing retreat with student seminars, and a diverse range of scholars interacting with students' thesis committees. But achieving transdisciplinarity is not without challenges. Working together in a transdisciplinary way is difficult because participating trainees and mentors are often overwhelmed by the amount of information in everyday practice and because of the incommensurability of specialized languages and definitons in each of the fields of expertise.

The training of student researchers and scholars in CPHR is transdisciplinary for at least three reasons. First, the range of health-determining conditions encompasses fields of inquiry spanning many different disciplines (e.g., social epidemiology, sociology, social work, geography, anthropology, political science, economics, environmental sciences). Different disciplines have given greater attention to different levels of these health-determining conditions, but no one discipline has encompassed all of the aspects necessary for a full understanding of what makes people healthy or sick at the population and societal levels. Second, each discipline offers differing theories or organizational schema for understanding these conditions and how they (or differing levels of social organization) interrelate or influence one another to produce health. Transdisciplinary research is necessary to integrate different disciplinary approaches into new ways of understanding how research questions might be framed in the first place. Third, each discipline employs or emphasizes different research methods, and therefore transdisciplinary research holds the possibility of enriching the depth and rigour of any particular study, or set of studies, by utilizing and triangulating among a number of different research methods and methodological approaches.

The second element in CPHR, the importance of *knowledge translation and exchange as a core competency for modern researchers*, demands that research also needs to be linked to policy sectors in ways that do not constrain the questions that might be posed, but ensure that research findings are immediately transferred into policy fields and discourses. Population health research is a practical undertaking that seeks to understand the conditions that create the greatest health for the greatest number. One of the challenges researchers face is moving their research findings beyond the publications that advance individual careers into the policy and practice arenas where decisions are made affecting population health-determining conditions. Learning how to do this as part of their training will make it easier for future generations of population health researchers to bridge the gap between research and policy.

The student researcher needs a good grounding in civil society partnerships. Future researchers need to be methodologically competent, with a deep understanding of theory, but also community savvy. Many poorer communities or population groups facing health-compromising conditions are frustrated with "being researched to death" or being subjected to "tokenism." They are demanding more active participation with researchers in framing questions, interpreting results, and disseminating findings, as well as holding researchers and their work accountable for the benefits it provides to people and not simply to academic careers. Research funding bodies are increasingly demanding evidence of such partnerships, but there is a risk of tokenism unless the power and cross-cultural dynamics of the research/policy/community sector triad are well understood and respectfully negotiated. This understanding and respect can be learned but not taught. It requires "learning by doing" in which researchers, community members, and policy-makers practice collaboration on specific research projects. CPHR has striven to inculcate these competencies in the students and trainees in the program.

The third element of CPHR, *strong mentorship*, is what makes the training experience for faculty and students a success. CPHR mentors go beyond the student-supervisor relationship; while mentors do act as advisors and role models, on a personal level they have also become teachers and friends to their students. The mentor relationship in the CPHR program offers an alternative to more formal hierarchies and structures in which both students and their academic mentors can freely exchange ideas and knowledge. Mentors serve as sounding boards and aid student development where they will themselves become inclined to take on mentoring roles in their own careers.

Continuing the SPHERU brand of research and mentorship, which is to produce new transdisciplinary knowledge in population health that is both relevant and compelling for researchers and communities within Saskatchewan and elsewhere, remains an important goal within SPHERU's mandate.

SETTING NEW DIRECTIONS IN POPULATION HEALTH RESEARCH

The essays collected here, as noted above, were originally presented at a joint SPHERU—CPHR conference held in Saskatchewan in autumn 2008 and represent the kind of population health research that SPHERU and CPHR endeavour both to promote and to produce. The collection represents new voices in the field. The essays employ new methods, use traditional methodologies in new ways, present new theoretical perspectives, and challenge existing perspectives; they examine or propose new or different interventions as means of reducing health inequalities and highlight new ways of thinking about how research links to policy and practice in reducing those inequalities.

The first section of this volume deals with theoretical, conceptual, and ethical issues raised around how we understand critical population health research as an essentially political project. Guerrero's paper, "The Essential Value(s) of Health: Implications for Canadian Population Health Research and Policy," poses a fundamental question for population health researchers when he argues that the measurement of success of programs and policies will ultimately rest on how we understand health. He reviews several prominent definitions of health for their appropriateness within a population health approach and concludes that these definitions generally lack conceptual clarity and are too broad in scope. Guerrero argues for a balance between a naturalist and normativist view of how we understand health, challenges us to make explicit the values that are embedded within current population health research and policy, and further advocates for agreement on a minimal account of health that will address the reduction of health disparities more directly.

The paper by Abonyi and a number of her SPHERU colleagues, "Towards an Ethical Framework for Population Health Research in Canada: A Place for Ethical Space?," explores the notion of creating ethical space as a means of accommodating differences in world views held by researchers and the subjects of research. It is through a process of dialogue between researchers and the communities with whom they engage in research that one can develop different approaches to research that break down the traditional researcher-subject dichotomy and begin to develop truly collaborative partnerships. The work of Ermine and Pimple provides a foundation upon which the authors argue for a restructuring of the research process rooted in a dialogue that seeks common ground between often very different epistemological positions. This leads to an engagement between researchers and the communities they work with that sees those communities as true partners in the research process and provides those communities with tools with which to confront the health inequalities they face.

The paper by Nowatzki, "Income Inequality and Health: A Theoretical Quagmire," provides a much-needed overview of the theoretical perspectives underlying the burgeoning income inequality–population health research. One of the advances or shifts in thinking that occurred in the mid-1990s with the ascendancy of population health (first in Canada and elsewhere later) is the firm understanding of the powerful contribution of unequal income distribution to the health of populations. This story was more than merely income-poor people being sicker than income-rich people. A decade and half ago researchers in the United Kingdom and elsewhere showed conclusively that income and health are related in a gradient way and that, at a population level, average income gains fail to buy increasing levels of health beyond a certain threshold. These deep understandings about how we are all affected by unequal income distributions have recently been somewhat compromised by the ascendancy, once again, of the poverty argument. Nowatzki's paper is not only timely in that it may rebalance the discourse now seemingly dominated by "poverty research," but also because it provides much-needed possible explanations for how living in a society with great income inequalities affects peoples' health.

The second section focuses on challenging some of the traditional understandings of population health policy by offering critical reassessments of some important issues that challenge long-held assumptions. In examining the tragic and oft-reported phenomenon of high suicide rates amongst Aboriginal youth in Canada, Teucher's paper, "Aboriginal Health Research and Epidemiology: Differences between Indigenous and Western Knowledge," presents important qualifications not only in how we perceive the issue itself, but also in how we conceptualize and think about differences between Aboriginal and non-Aboriginal ways of knowing. Teucher argues that non-Aboriginal researchers and governments fail to acknowledge that some solutions to social problems in Aboriginal communities may exist within Aboriginal communities, rooted within Indigenous epistemologies and cultural expressions that are too often denied or ignored by the dominant society. The challenge, then, is first to allow Indigenous ways of knowing to have a voice in order to understand what makes specific Indigenous communities healthy, but also to understand that there are multiple epistemological standpoints between different Indigenous communities and peoples and that the transfer of knowledge and experience between Aboriginal communities is neither straightforward nor linear.

Chessie's discussion of the role of citizen governors within the health system provides a timely assessment of some of the long-held assumptions about how best to move the health system's focus towards a greater emphasis on prevention, health promotion, and health determinants. "The Shifting Discourse of 'Public Participation': Implications in Changing Models of Health System Regionalization" demonstrates that enhanced and higher profile roles for citizen governors were a key element of the regionalization of provincial health systems, which were intended to help break down the traditional focus on institutions and acute care as the *sine qua non* of health care. Using Saskatchewan's two waves of regionalization reform, Chessie points to fundamental flaws in the manner in which the role of citizen governors, and especially their role in facilitating greater democratic input and control of decision-making, has been conceptualized and operationalized. The end result is not to abandon the idea of public participation but to rethink its goals and its implementation in a manner that can account for the competing logics that surround it.

The final paper in this section, Hippe's "A Healthy Pregnancy is in Your Hands," offers important contributions for two distinct, but related, reasons. Hippe offers some fresh insights on pregnancy and health by contextualizing women's experiences of prenatal care within a social and medical care system and women's agency. Hippe's paper sits at the intersections of maternal/child health, gender and health, health care services, epidemiology, social theory, and public policy. In this way, the paper advances the cause of transdisciplinary research that integrates knowledge from multiple disciplinary perspectives, rebalances the predominance of quantitative and positivist methodology in maternal/child health research, and lets the reader in closer to the real world of women experiencing pregnancy in our society.

The third and final section focuses on some very specific population health interventions and issues that provide important insights into how one might reconsider alternative interventions in the future. Shaw discusses the application of a population health perspective through presentation of a study exploring the role of dragon boat racing as a source of social and emotional support for women experiencing breast cancer. "Dragon Boat Racing as an Alternative Type of Support for Women Living with Breast Cancer" highlights the point that gendered inequalities influence the social relationships and cultural practices that shape women's experiences of leisure and organized support. The findings from her study suggest the importance of alternatives to traditional forms of breast cancer support. Effective support interventions would recognize both the range of needs of women experiencing breast cancer and the structured inequalities that pervade women's lives.

Bowen and Muhajarine provide an example of the practice of integrating population health perspective with different levels of intervention and prevention when working with pregnant women experiencing depression. "Integrating Population Health Promotion and Prevention: A Model Approach to Research and Action for Vulnerable Pregnant Women" summarizes the effects of depression in pregnancy on the fetus and growing child and highlights the effectiveness of specific interventions, but argues that it is also important to understand the health determinants associated with antenatal depression. Their study highlights the value of a population health perspective, particularly in terms of promoting primary prevention and the ability to direct services and interventions to those women who are affected most by the context of social inequalities. Their integrated model of prevention and population health guided their research activities and, in turn, facilitated knowledge translation activities and the development of new programming.

The final paper in the volume, Cushon and Muhajarine's "The Cousin of Globalization: Neo-liberalism and Child-Relevant Policy," examines the local impact of globalization and its cousin, neo-liberalism. Whereas most traditional examinations of the health impacts of economic, political, and cultural globalization focus on state-level impacts, this essay offers a unique view into how these processes have changed domestic policy outcomes that themselves changed the health landscape of a mid-sized Canadian city (in this case, Saskatoon, SK).

Of particular concern to the authors is how neo-liberalism in Canada was expressed relative to child-relevant policy outcomes at the local, provincial, and national level. Greater reliance on market mechanisms, significant attempts to off-load responsibility to other orders of government, and a stronger emphasis on individual rather than collective responsibility—all hallmarks of neo-liberal economic and social policy—have reshaped child policy amongst all orders of government. What remains uncertain is whether the social investment strategy employed in elements of this new policy landscape will yield the health benefits its proponents hold for it.

FINAL THOUGHTS

The papers presented here, and the conference from which they originated, are really only the starting point for a sustained discussion about "new directions" for population health research in Canada. They cover a broad range of subjects from the theoretical and conceptual through to the challenges of policy-making and the evaluation of interventions. However, they are indicative of the kinds of critical, self-reflexive, and normative research that lies at the heart of the political project that is population health research. The goal of this volume is to contribute to that project and, perhaps, to add some new dimensions to it by giving voice to newer research and researchers who sometimes have a difficult time being heard.

REFERENCES

Bramley, D., Herbert, P., Tuzzio, L., & Chassin, M. (2005). Disparities in Indigenous health: A cross-country comparison between New Zealand and the United States. *American Journal of Public Health, 95*(5), 844–850.

DesMeules, M., & Pong, R. (2006). *How healthy are rural Canadians? An assessment of their health status and health determinants.* Ottawa: Canadian Institute for Health Information.

Dressler, W. W., & Bindon, J. R. (2000). The health consequences of cultural consonance: Cultural dimensions of lifestyle, social support, and arterial blood pressure in an African American community. *American Anthropologist, 102*(2), 244–260.

Dressler, W. W., Oths, K. S, & Gravlee, C. C. (2005). Race and ethnicity in public health research: Models to explain health disparities. *Annual Review of Anthropology, 34,* 231–268.

Jebamani, L. S., Burchill, C. A., & Martens, P. J. (2005). Using data linkage to identify First Nations Manitobans. *Canadian Journal of Public Health, 96*(Suppl 1), S28-S32.

Jeffery, B., Abonyi, S., Labonte, R., & Duncan, K. (2006). Engaging numbers: Health indicators that matter for people, place and practice. *Journal of Aboriginal Health, 3*(1), 44–52.

Johnson, S., Abonyi, S., Jeffery, B., Hackett, P., Hampton, M., McIntosh, T., Martz, D., Muhajarine, N., Petrucka, P., & Sari, N. (2008). Recommendations for action on the social determinants of health—A Canadian perspective. *The Lancet* (UK), 372, 1690–1693.

Kingdon, J. W. ([1995] 2003). *Agendas, alternatives and public policies* (2nd Ed.). New York: Addison-Wesley Educational Publishers Inc.

Kingdon, J. W. (2006). The reality of public policy making. In M. Danis, C.M. Clancy, and L.R. Churchill (Eds.), *Ethical dimensions of health policy* (pp. 97–116). Oxford: Oxford University Press.

Labonte, R., Polanyi, M., Muhajarine, N., Mcintosh, M., & Williams, A. 2005. Beyond the divides: Towards critical population health research. *Critical Public Health 15*(1), 5–17.

Martz, D., & Sanderson, K. (2006). The economic and social contribution of the public sector to rural Saskatchewan. *Journal of Rural and Community Development 1*(2). Retrieved from http://www.jrcd.ca/viewarticle.php?id=52

Martz, D., Reed, M., Brueckner, I., & Mills, S. (2006). *Hidden actors, muted voices: The employment of rural women in Saskatchewan forestry and agri-food industries.* Ottawa, ON: Status of Women Canada.

Nicolescu, B. (Ed.). (2008). *Transdisciplinarity—Theory and practice.* Cresskill, NJ: Hampton Press.

Romanow, R. J. (2002). *Building on values: The future of health care in Canada—final report.* [Saskatoon]: Commission on the Future of Health Care in Canada, November 2002.

Saskatchewan Health (2004). *Saskatchewan: Healthy people, a healthy province. Health research strategy.* Regina, SK: Saskatchewan Health.

Sinclair, R., Smith, R., & Stevenson, N. (2006). *Miyo-Mahcihowin: A report on Indigenous health in Saskatchewan.* Indigenous Peoples Health Research Centre: First Nations University of Canada, University of Saskatchewan & University of Regina.

Smylie, J., & Anderson, M. (2006). Understanding the health of Indigenous peoples in Canada: Key methodological and conceptual challenges. *Canadian Medical Association Journal, 175*(6), 602–605.

Wilson, K., & Rosenberg, M. W. (2002). Exploring the determinants of health for First Nations peoples in Canada: Can existing frameworks accommodate traditional activities? *Social Science and Medicine, 55,* 2017–2031.

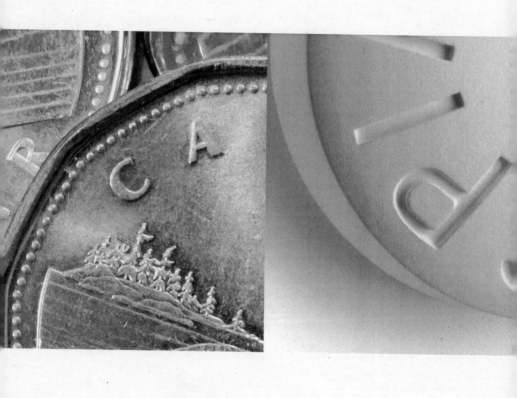

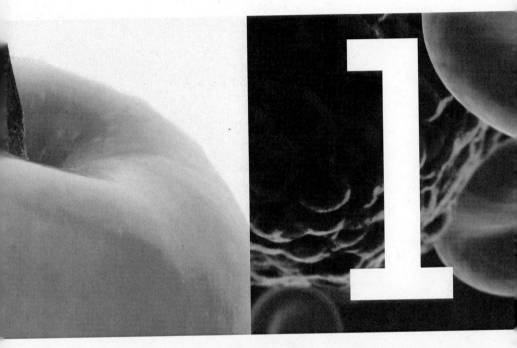

1

THEORY AND ETHICS

The Essential Value(s) of Health: Implications for Canadian Population Health Research and Policy

J. David Guerrero

INTRODUCTION

The prominence of the population health approach reflects a shift in our understanding of "health" as the absence of disease, a negative concept, to that of a capacity or resource, a positive concept. One result of this shift should be the recognition that which account of health a population health approach *ought* to employ is an important and substantive issue. After all, would it not be a mistake to make the capacity to hold one's breath under water for eight minutes a requirement for health? Another result of this shift should be the acknowledgment of the pressing need to be as clear as possible about the account of health that is, in fact, being employed to underpin population health research and policy. A clear understanding of *what the operational view of health is* is needed because, roughly put, different views of health will surely lead to the advancement of different strategies, different determinants, different outcomes, and different populations measured to be in greater or lesser health. Indeed, it is difficult to overstate the claim that tremendous consequences, for both society and the individuals deemed "unhealthy," turns on how we understand health. *A fortiori*, a population health approach would be remiss to understate the demands that change with the shift in our understanding of health.

The substantial point is that a *responsible* population health approach will recognize and acknowledge that:

1. The means for realizing the goals of "healthy people and healthy communities" are inevitably a function of what we understand "health(y)" to be;
2. We *ought* to insist that the best understanding of health be employed to underpin current—and future—Canadian population health research and policy.

Thus, a responsible population health approach will champion the call for employing the best understanding of health, taking a proactive role in determining what we understand health to be.[1]

So how do we understand health? The World Health Organization (WHO) gives arguably the most well-known account of health. The WHO constitution states that health is "a state of complete physical, mental, and social well-being and not merely the absence of disease or infirmity" (WHO, 1946, p. 2). This positive view of health has been a matter of significant controversy, and I believe rightly so. To its credit, Health Canada (1998) recognized that a profound problem with the WHO definition of health was that in "making health synonymous with well-being... [the WHO] confused health with its determinants and made it unmeasurable as the outcome of action addressing those determinants" (p. 7). Indeed, nearly 12 years later, one can find this *exact* sentiment on the Public Health Agency of Canada (PHAC) website; presumably, this is because the PHAC continues to deem the WHO definition of health inadequate to underpin Canadian population health research and policy. In light of this, the following statement is surely striking, if not altogether puzzling:

> In a manner consistent with the World Health Organization's definition of health as a state of complete physical, mental and social well-being and not merely the absence of disease, the Agency focuses on promoting health and minimizing the extent and impact of infectious and chronic diseases, injuries and emergencies. (PHAC, 2007, pp. 14–15)

Now, given all that has been stated, a reasonable person might legitimately wonder, first, if the PHAC is employing the best account of health possible and, second, if there is good reason to think that the current account(s) of health employed by the PHAC may also be inadequate to underpin a Canadian population health approach. Such thinking would be correct—or so I shall now argue.

In section 2, in order to advance my argument, I draw out two serious problems that a population health approach should have with the WHO definition of health. In section 3, I contend that the force of these problems strikes against the account(s) of "health" one currently finds in notable Canadian population health literature. In section 4, I propose we turn to a philosophical conception of health, and I argue that the best account of "health" to underpin population health will be essentially buttressed by human values. In section 5, I conclude with a discussion of some of the implications a value-laden account of health has for Canadian population health research and policy and suggest some strategies for change.

THE WHO DEFINITION OF HEALTH: TWO SIGNIFICANT PROBLEMS

The first problem is that the WHO definition simply lacks the requisite conceptual clarity to guide population health. An immediate worry is that the standard for health is set so high that nobody is—or likely will ever be—healthy. If, however, some people are in fact healthy, then we need to know what "a state of complete physical, mental and social well-being" actually amounts to, in order to sensibly distinguish healthy populations from unhealthy ones. But this raises a number of highly contentious issues that extend far beyond our present scope. For one, it requires that we be reasonably agreed upon who is going to determine the criteria for the "complete states" of well-being. Will such states vary from individual to individual depending upon the wants and desires one may happen to have? If so, opposing views of what "a complete state of well-being" properly entails will virtually guarantee different scopes and goals for a population health approach. Perhaps it might be asserted that a complete state of well-being in some important sense should be based on "objective" criteria. But given that we do have opposing wants and desires, it is not clear on what grounds one would legitimately favour the well-being—and, as such, the health—of *some* over the well-being and health of *others*. These are important issues that must be addressed (elsewhere!). Let us merely note that the vagueness of the WHO definition is a challenge for formulating any sort of principled standard that everyone would accept as constituting health.

The second problem is that the WHO definition of health is far too broad. According to Mordacci and Sobel (1998), if the WHO definition is taken literally, then it is meaningless. In the philosophy of health literature, the most common kinds of criticisms have centred on the way in which health is made to include nearly all of well-being: these criticisms typically proceed by providing grounds for believing that the WHO definition is too inclusive because it erroneously embraces *any* alleged criteria of well-being as integral components of health—criteria, for instance, such as achieving happiness (Kass, 1981, pp. 5–6), finding a four-leaf clover (Richman, 2004, pp. 27–61), realizing an IQ of 400 (Stark, 2006, p. 59), and improving poor Internet connections, etc. There is a serious problem lurking here for a population health approach. To appreciate the force of the problem, it is worth explicitly noting that the two standard objectives of population health are to improve the health of the entire population and to reduce health inequalities among population groups (PHAC, 2009).[2] Now, if we take these objectives seriously (as a responsible population health approach surely must), then the broadness of the WHO definition sets counterintuitive targets for population health. For example, even if improved Internet connections would increase the overall social well-being for Canadians, it is surely a mistaken account of health that would compel one to identify, say, Internet connection speeds to be a determinant of health and, what is more, to devote resources to reduce Internet speed disparities among Canadians.[3] In the population health literature, as noted above, powerful criticisms are directed against the inability of the WHO definition to distinguish between health and well-being. Frankish et al. (1996) echo this objection and further report that a prevalent line of criticism raised against such all-encompassing views of health is that they are "hopelessly utopian and infeasible" (p. 6). For our purposes, the point to press is that a satisfactory account of health will distinguish "health" in some sense from what simply might reasonably—or unreasonably!—be thought to contribute to one's well-being. This will require our operational account of health to have a significant amount of conceptual clarity and precision.

HEALTH: A CANADIAN PERSPECTIVE

It follows from this that we should want to be sure that a Canadian population health approach does not employ an operational account of health that clearly lacks the requisite amount of conceptual clarity and precision. After all, we should not want Canadian population health research and policy to be guided by a flawed understanding of health. To that end, an investigation is in order. Here it is important to pause and note two things: first, there are several very different accounts of health that seem to be in operation and, second, for obvious reasons, I can discuss only a few here.

Keeping these two points in mind, an obvious place to start is with the Public Health Agency of Canada. On their website, one can find a promising heading entitled "Population Health: Defining Health." Here we are told that there has been a shift in the thinking of the population health approach such that it no longer embraces the WHO definition of health and that:

> [t]he population health approach recognizes that health is a capacity or resource rather than a state, a definition which corresponds more to the notion of being able to pursue one's goals, to acquire skills and education, and to grow. (PHAC, 2009)

But is this definition of health better equipped to overcome the two serious problems that stand against the WHO definition? It might be claimed that an important difference is the explicit claim that health is to be conceptualized in terms of a capacity and an ability to act rather than merely a state. Perhaps this makes explicit how we often speak of health in ordinary language and maybe even better facilitates a population health approach, but this alone hardly adds the requisite conceptual clarity that a population health approach surely demands. We saw that a serious problem with the WHO definition of health is that it is too inclusive, but it is difficult to see how "the notion of being able to pursue one's goals, to acquire skills and education, and to grow" is in and of itself necessarily more limiting. After all, is it immediately obvious why one's goal could not be to grow into a state of complete physical, mental, and social well-being? Surely not. Thus, to think the problems that strike against the WHO definition are turned away by simply stipulating that health is a capacity or resource is erroneous.

In order to avoid an unfair characterization, it is important to note that after stating that their adopted definition of health recognizes the various broad factors that impact health, the PHAC, following Frankish et al. (1996), goes on to state: The best articulation of this concept of health is "the capacity of people to adapt to, respond to, or control life's challenges and changes" (PHAC 2009).[4] Framing health as a capacity in terms of "life's challenges and changes" is an improvement up to a point; it does, I think, serve to limit the broadness of health to some extent, but exactly to what extent is an open question. Presumably, it would serve to eliminate some unrealistic goals (e.g., for me to be the tallest Canadian) and implausible skills (e.g., time travel) from becoming a central component of health. And insofar as the goal to grow into a state of complete physical, mental, and social well-being could be considered to be unrealistic and/or implausible, then this view of health will be significantly more limiting than the WHO definition. But surely a reasonable person may wonder if it is still, in fact, too broad a view of health. After all, even a blind man who has just been poisoned and stabbed in the leg by a scorned lover and bitten in the other leg by a rabid dog has some capacity to respond to life's challenges and changes; yet I think no reasonable person would consider this man to be healthy. Thus, a qualification must be added: If we count an individual to be healthy, then we are maintaining that this individual possesses not just *any* capacity but some minimal capacity "to adapt to, respond to, or control life's challenges and changes." Although I think this qualification is palpable, it is important to be clear that, when it comes to formulating a minimal capacity of health, it is not at all obvious what criteria we should employ or even how to legitimately ground the choice of criteria. Thus, in many instances it will be an open question whether or not to count an individual or population healthy.

Nevertheless, we do, in fact, count people and populations to be unhealthy. And to the extent that we do so, we surely must be employing some notion of a minimal standard of health. In light of this, surely a reasonable person might wonder what exactly the capacity to adapt to, respond to, or control is—either implicitly or explicitly—since it is deemed a requirement to being "healthy." This is especially so given that, as I noted above, exactly what minimal capacity we should employ is such an important and substantive issue. And, what is more, it may have different answers, depending upon one's particular agenda.

Another view of health can be found in Health Canada's *The Population Health Template: Key Elements and Actions that Define a Population Health Approach* (2001). Here, we find one notable difference in that the authors explicitly state both (a) their view of health and (b) that their view of health provides the foundation for their understanding of the population health approach. The claim, in short, is that a Canadian population health approach rests ultimately on the following understanding of health: "Health is a capacity or resource for everyday living that enables us to pursue our goals, acquire skills and education, grow, and satisfy personal aspirations" (Health Canada, 2001, p. 2).[5] This definition is an upgrade at least insofar as "everyday living" may be persuasively thought to serve as some sort of limiting criteria. But this definition of health is still far from being satisfactory because it fails to make explicit with the requisite clarity and precision the criteria for determining health and, as such, ill health. For example: To what extent must we have a capacity or resource to be satisfactorily "enabled" to pursue *our* goals and acquire skills and education? Is there a principled standard of "everyday living" or will it vary from individual to individual and/or population to population? If it is the former, then who sets it? And if it is the latter, then, given that different views of "everyday living" will demand the satisfaction of different levels of skills, education, and growth that will surely require different capacities or resources, it is difficult to see how this conception of health would not, in fact, perpetuate some "health" inequalities. After all, different people do in fact want different—and crucially opposing—"goals" and "personal aspirations" satisfied. And if this were the case, then a serious worry would be that *any* whim, unrealistic goal, or fiat could demarcate health. A related and very serious worry here is that it might be claimed that we can improve the overall health of a population if we were to have them, say, set different or lower standards when it comes to "*their* goals and personal aspirations."

In sum, all of the above accounts of health have left us with open questions (to which many more could be added) with serious practical implications—not the least of which is who will and who will not count as healthy—that demand explicit answers. Unless and until these questions are answered, a population health approach that builds upon any one of the above accounts of health builds upon a dubious foundation that, at best, lacks principled grounds to prefer the scope and goals of one view over another when faced with conflicting population health research and policy and, at worst, enables health to become a social engineering control of a population's behaviour.[6] This realization motivates a pressing need to talk about the account of health that *ought* to be employed. Because we require a better understanding of *what health is*, I propose we turn to a philosophical conception of health.

THE PHILOSOPHY OF HEALTH: THE MODERN DEBATE

There are two major positions in the philosophy of health literature: naturalism and normativism. Naturalists contend that "health" is both an empirically and an objectively discernible concept. The alleged upshot of the naturalist's "realist" account is that "health" has a theoretical foundation in value-free science. Normativists contend that "health" is an inextricably value-laden concept—a healthy population is necessarily connected to a human value choice.

Insofar as the concept of health is value-laden, then, ultimately so too is the concept of population health itself *if* population health is to be understood as an approach to improving overall health and reducing health disparities. *A fortiori*, insofar as science *qua* science can be thought to be strictly a value-neutral pursuit, we may have to concede that population health lacks a scientific foundation. This should provide a strong motivation to take the naturalist position seriously. To my mind, Arthur Caplan (1993) nicely emphasizes why many are keen to resist a normativist concept of health and disease when he says: "The greater the role of values in the definition of health and disease, the worse the prognosis appears to be for both their objectivity and reality" (pp. 240–241). A common criticism of normativism is that without a value-free epistemic foundation we may ultimately have no principled grounds to prefer the scope and goals of one conception of health and disease over another. This is an understandable concern given that so many of us want to say that it was and is wrong to classify homosexuality, masturbation, and "drapetomania"—the condition that caused slaves to run away from their masters—as "diseases." Concerning himself solely with empirically observable facts, the naturalist claims to sidestep these mistaken classifications, which are perceived as dangerous possibilities when values are introduced into the account of health.

9

The Biostatistical Theory (BST)

The most influential "naturalist" account of health and disease is Christopher Boorse's biostatistical theory (BST).[7] The BST is a complex theory that Boorse has developed in several papers over many years (Boorse, 1975, 1976, 1977, 1987, 1997, 2002). Given the scope of this paper, we must concern ourselves with only a very brief sketch of Boorse's view of health. Nevertheless, it is one that I submit will suffice to convincingly show that the BST, as it is currently conceived, is unfit to underpin a responsible population health approach. However, in order to gloss over many of the complexities of the BST, let us grant from the outset that the BST does, in fact, advance value-free concepts of health and disease.[8] With this in mind, Boorse (1997) has most recently advanced the following official definitions:

> The *reference class* is a natural class of organisms of uniform functional design, specifically, an age group of a sex of a species.

> A *normal function* of a part or process within members of the reference class is a statistically typical contribution by it to their *individual* survival and reproduction.

> A *disease* is a type of internal state which is either an impairment of normal functional ability, i.e., a reduction of one or more functional abilities below typical efficiency, or a limitation on functional ability caused by environmental agents.

> *Health* is the absence of disease. (pp.7–8)[9]

To his credit, Boorse offers an explicit definition of "disease," and when one takes seriously his official definition schema it would seem he commits the BST to the following positive definition of health: an individual is healthy if and only if *all* the functions that contribute to the individual's survival and reproduction *today* are capable of performing in a way that is species-typical (i.e., the *statistical norm* of the relevant functions of the same species, sex, and age at time *t*) on species-typical occasions.

There are two points worth explicitly noting. First, Boorse (1997, p. 28) firmly insists that the only functions *relevant* to the determination of health are those that contribute to individual survival and reproduction.[10] This is a very contentious claim since, of course, that would suggest that discomfort (e.g., shingles, carpal tunnel syndrome) and inconvenience (e.g., high arch foot, Raynaud's disease) of functioning as well as the capacity to achieve a quality of life (e.g., education, income, and social status) are not to be counted relevant considerations of health unless, even in a modern society, they contribute to individual survival and reproduction success.[11] This becomes a substantive issue given the multifarious health determinants that are advanced in notable population health literature. For example, in identifying education as a health determinant the Canadian Senate states that "[e]ducation can increase income and job security, and give people a sense of control over their life circumstances—key factors in good health" (Senate of Canada, 2008b, p. 4). Suffice to say that for anyone to insist that determinants of health extend beyond the BST's twin desiderata of individual survival and reproduction means their view of health will not solely be the BST.

There is another, especially persuasive, reason for a responsible population health approach not to accept Boorse's BST, which brings us to the second point worth noting. Recall that health is to be conceived of entirely in terms of biological processes (function) and statistics (normality of function). Correspondingly, the minimal standard for health is underwritten, first and foremost, by "species-typical functioning." What is to be stressed is that health-status ultimately becomes tantamount to statistical average functioning that may fluctuate given changes in the data collected from the reference class. The problem with this, from a population health perspective, is that the minimal standard of health will be dynamic and may change as the various individuals who presently form the various reference classes change individually, or as the membership of the reference class changes. To understand why this is so troubling one needs only to realize that a significant increase in "health disparities" between populations could, in fact, lead to an overall decrease in the minimum standard of health such that more—and not fewer!—individuals would count as being "healthy." Surely a population health approach that would, for example, intentionally seek to increase inequalities between or amongst populations in order to count individuals as "healthy" is not merely factually wrong-headed; it is unjust.

The cost of employing the BST's value-free minimal standard of health runs higher still and may be introduced as follows: If one accepts the framework of the BST, then health becomes wedded to what is statistically normal for a reference class. However, statistically normal functioning is not and should not be deemed a sufficient condition for health. It is not a sufficient condition for health because, simply put, an unhealthy individual can be functioning, statistically speaking, normally. Even if all humans were to become grossly obese, there would still be people functioning at or above what is statistically speaking "normal"; yet insofar as gross obesity clearly threatens an individual's ability, we should surely not want to count such people as healthy.[12] And once we realize that the framework of the BST is such that the statistical norms the BST crucially advances only mark how we are in fact functioning, it becomes clear that what essentially matters for health is not and should not be statistically normal functioning. There is simply no guarantee that how we do, in fact, function is how we *ought* to be functioning or even that we are functioning well. This realization brings to light a significant hidden cost that comes with adopting Boorse's BST. That is, insofar as disparities in health are thought to negatively impact an individual's relevant functioning, then what the BST ultimately counts to be "statistically normal functioning" will clearly be determined in part by existing health inequalities and, what is most troubling, by existing health inequities. Indeed, a fundamental problem with the BST's minimal standard of health is that it hopelessly interweaves "health" and "health inequities." To be sure, if we adopt the BST's value-free minimal standard of health, we will be compelled to promote and perpetuate the very health disparities a population health approach surely seeks to reduce. This is a price that a responsible population health approach cannot afford to pay.

The preceding shows that the two standard objectives of population health crucially run against the BST's minimal standard of health. It must be stressed, then, that the BST should not be considered fit to solely underpin a responsible population health approach. And so long as the BST remains the leading naturalist account of health one ought to insist that the best account of health to underpin a population health approach will be inextricably value-laden. How much comfort can be taken in the claim that Boorse's BST is unsuitable to underpin population health? Considerable comfort can be found not so much on the rejection of naturalism's main contender—for there could conceivably be better naturalist offerings toeing the line—but in the force of the rejection. Indeed, it seems plausible to say that we are rejecting the most promising naturalist conception of biological fitness. After all, ultimately what is being rejected is health being defined in terms of evolutionary biological fitness, that is, statistically normal biological functioning. In any case, if there is a better naturalist account of health waiting in the wings, then it ought to be put forth. Unless and until this is done, we must acknowledge that a responsible population health approach will employ an account of health that is essentially based—implicitly or explicitly—on human values.[13] So let's turn to normativism and look at what this may imply for our understanding of health.

Normativism: A Very Brief Word
The normativist maintains that the explicit reference to human values enables his framework to square with our intuitions that health is a more robust state of being than his naturalist counterpart allows for. For population health

research and policy, an obvious appeal of the normativist framework is that it is not constrained by the BST's twin desiderata of individual survival and reproduction. This is clearly a compelling advantage of normativism. However, matters become much more complex when we take seriously what a commitment to normativism further implies for our understanding of health. The literature neatly distinguishes normativism from naturalism, but it is by no means clear exactly what the implications are for our understanding of health from the decision to opt for a normativist conception.

At least part of the problem is that different implications will arise depending upon one's preferred normativist conception of health—and there is no shortage of these to choose from. The normativist side is well represented by diverse value-laden theories, such as Fulford's (1989) "reverse view"; Nordenfelt's (1987, 2004) "welfare theory"; Pörn's (1993) "equilibrium model"; and Richman's (2004) "embedded instrumentalist" theory of health. Although these theorists are united in their agreement that a viable conception of health must reference values, there is fierce disagreement not only over what these requisite values are to be, but also over what empirical facts regarding health are relevant and to what extent, if at all, these facts are to be value-driven. For our purposes, what is to be stressed is that there is a real sense in which theorists take normativism to be a crucially abstract receptacle in which to couch quite different—and often opposing—sorts of content. For the normativist, a significant problem is to persuasively articulate what a *well-grounded* normativist understanding of health would be. Indeed, all of the accounts of health examined in section 3 notably failed to satisfactorily articulate crucial content—content (e.g., "the notion of being able to pursue one's goals"; "capacity or resource for everyday living") that, it can hardly be denied, there are many plausible—and opposing—ways to interpret. The lesson a population approach should take from this is that a deeper understanding of health is in order. To that end, there is an antecedent need to become clearer about the fundamental differences among normativists within the modern debate. How we negotiate between opposing normativist claims carries profound implications not only for our understanding of health per se, but also for our understanding of population health research and policy.

For those of us concerned with strengthening population health research and policy, the recognition that an adequate account of the minimal functioning and/or capacity requisite for health *will* be crucially generated by human values provides the impetus for a significant encounter with normativism. No longer can we simply allow vague and ambiguous value-laden concepts to play an all-too-critical role in our operational account of health. Thus we must demand clarity and precision. It is important to be mindful that health, it does seem, is a paronymous concept with complex extensions that will not be defined by a crisp set of necessary and sufficient conditions. Nevertheless, the fact that there is a plurality of (opposing) values among different populations underscores the need to take very seriously Aristotle's (1984) call in the *Nicomachean Ethics* "to look for precision in each class of things just so far as the nature of the subject admits" (p. 1730).[14] To be sure, it will be extremely difficult to strike a balance between a comprehensive account of health and one that is sufficiently clear and precise to underpin population health research and policy. But no reasonable person should expect otherwise.

FURTHER IMPLICATIONS AND STRATEGIES FOR CHANGE

A commitment to normativism poses some important intellectual challenges for a population health approach—challenges that I believe have not received the attention they deserve.[15] For example, we need to become much clearer on what values—as well as whose—ought to play a fundamental role in responsible health judgements. A related need is to get a better idea of the role that values may (or may not) play in evaluations of health and of strategies that affect population health. Most importantly, considerable efforts should be given to making explicit the values that currently play an essential role in Canadian population health research and practice. To be sure, these challenges are not just the theoretical fare of philosophers and health theorists: If we want to be sure the concept of health we employ does not, in fact, perpetuate the very health disparities we supposedly seek to reduce, then we need to keep a clear idea of the value(s) of "health" that can and do underpin Canadian population health. After all, it is not at all obvious that Canadian health policy-makers believe that social, political, and economic inequalities are ipso facto bad.

The reluctance of those concerned with population health to confront the challenges of normativism enable questionable accounts of health to underpin current Canadian population health initiatives—accounts that allow health disparities between populations to remain stubbornly resistant to change. I have tried to show that a significant problem with the accounts of health purporting to underpin population health is the lack of clarity and precision. The fact that we can readily shape opposing values into vague and ambiguous accounts of health should, it seems to me, serve to underscore this point. This is a point that cannot be overstated. By relying upon ambiguous, value-laden notions, in the face of all the identified determinants of health and the increasing persistence of both health inequalities and inequities—and notwithstanding its explicit mandate to reduce health disparities—Canadian population health research and policy allows an avenue for people to advance values that participate in the matrix of discrimination and oppression. Simply put, ambiguous content significantly undermines the ability to achieve the stipulated population health objectives. Thus, we announce a mandate to reduce health inequalities among population groups. Furthermore, we observe and measure that income and social status are determinants of health and we proclaim that poverty perpetuates ill health. Yet, we crucially lack a substantive claim as to what reducing socio-economic *health disparities* reasonably entails. This is a profound shortcoming because, for better or for worse, creating a more equitable distribution of money and resources requires considerable justification. Consequently, without a persuasive claim about what reducing socio-economic *health disparities* reasonably entails, there is a real sense that there is nothing tangible for a responsible population health approach to dig its teeth into that would compel positive change. In practice, we are well-intentioned but toothless. The inability to translate knowledge into action has not gone unnoticed by some; the Senate of Canada (2008a) aptly describes our dismal practical impact:

> Sadly, the great majority of those fine policy statements that have been produced by the federal, provincial and territorial governments since the Lalonde report, 30 years ago, to foster greater emphasis on the non-medical determinants of health, population health, and health disparities remain little more than well-meaning but empty rhetoric. Canadians deserve better! (p. 91)

Yet, less than five months in the wake of this Senate of Canada (2008a) report, the Canadian Public Health Association (CPHA) affirmed that "Canada can be proud of its overall health achievements" (CPHA, 2008, p. 5). This is especially disturbing because, after reporting that, of 30 countries surveyed, no country spends more money on health care to achieve worse results than Canada, the Senate of Canada (2008a) pulls no punches in stating "[t]hese sobering numbers tell us we are doing something terribly wrong regarding health and the health care delivery system" (p. 91). Simply put, we can no longer afford to mask this reality. We need to make it our business to demand that our operational account of health clearly and precisely (as much as possible) explicates the minimal standards requisite for health. Not only would this improve upon the failings of the above accounts of health, but it may also equip us with the needed teeth to significantly reduce health disparities among Canadians. For if one views health to be of special value such that it is something that every Canadian is in some sense entitled to as a matter of justice or morality, then insofar as our social policy choices perpetuate inequalities in health they could be considered to be unjust or morally wrong. We should take advantage of the fact that the Senate Subcommittee on Population Health has explicitly stated that "[h]ealth is a fundamental human need and, therefore, a basic human right" (Senate of Canada, 2008b, p. 10). But what exactly does this basic human right entail? Does it entail living in better conditions than Vancouver's Downtown East Side? Or is it not being exposed to the significant risk of unsafe drinking water, as 75 percent of First Nation communities are? (Christensen, 2006, p. 30). Making sense of what it means to say that health is a basic human right requires justifying a minimal standard of health.

Speaking to the issue of justification, those of us concerned with improving population health should take advantage of the fact that there are few "hot button issues" that seem to justify immediate action more than perceived threats to one's health. Most importantly, we should take advantage of the fact that the account of health we employ *is* essentially tied to human values. If, for instance, we find ourselves employing an account of health that does little more than express the entrenched interests of others, then we ought to take issue with the values that essentially buttress such an account. Accordingly, I suggest: 1) that we make explicit and challenge the value(s) of health that essentially underpin our present population health research and policy; and 2) that considerable efforts be given to explicating a minimum standard of health. To incite positive change, I suggest that a Canadian population health approach should aim to secure a minimal account of health that can legitimately aim to reduce health disparities, especially those rooted in discrimination and oppression.[16]

NOTES

1. Clearly, further elaboration and qualification is called for. However, for the present purposes, this is enough to distinguish a responsible population health approach from a population health approach that stands content to build upon a clearly inadequate understanding of health. Part of the idea here is that, given the tremendous practical implications involved, so many of us want to be able so say that it would be irresponsible not to employ the best understanding of health that could be employed; and, moreover, that we *should not* employ an understanding of health that clearly perpetuates health disparities.

2. This two-fold objective is stated in several notable publications. See, for instance, the Senate of Canada (2008b, p. 3); and Health Canada (1998, p. 1).

3. It is important to be clear that nothing turns on my choice to use Internet connection speeds to illustrate the problem. The crux of the problem is that the WHO definition will compel a population health approach to ameliorate *any* alleged criterion of well-being— be it ill-fitting clothes; homesickness; the length and intensity of Canadian winters; or....

4. This exact wording also appears in Health Canada (1998, p. 7). See also Frankish et al. (1996, p. 6).

5. This view of health is also stated in Health Canada (1998, p. 7).

6. To illustrate: consider the Soviet-era practice to revise definitions of mental illness such that political dissidents were deemed mentally ill and, as such, forcibly detained in mental institutions. Unfortunately, this may not be a thing of the past as several notable news agencies have recently reported that Russia has revived this practice. To press this substantial point further: Lawrie Reznek (1987, pp. 6–8), remarks that there was a time when the desire for masturbation and homosexuality were each considered conditions that constitute disease and, most unfortunately for those individuals diagnosed with such "condition," the respective medical treatments were to cauterize the clitoris and burn out the part of the brain (the hypothalamus) thought responsible for homosexual behaviour.

7. See, for example, Cooper (2002), Nordenfelt (2004), Richman (2004), Khushf (2007), and Ereshefsky (2009).

8. A main line of criticism against the BST is that the resulting concepts of health and disease are inherently normative. To be sure, within the philosophy of biology literature it is a matter of significant controversy whether the biological concepts the BST employs are themselves value-free concepts. This is a matter that, for obvious reasons, cannot be explored here. However, it should be noted that for the BST to be no more normative than biology is surely all we should reasonably demand of Boorse.

9. I suspect many people will want to immediately reject Boorse's view of health just as soon as they learn that his official position is that "health is the absence of disease." But an outright rejection would be hasty—we ought to at least have a reasonably clear idea of Boorse's understanding of "disease." A fortiori, Khushf (1997) states: "Boorse's concept of disease clearly formulates a concept that is held by many (probably most) scientists and physicians, although they may not express it in the same manner or appreciate its implications" (p. 154).

10. Boorse (1997, p. 28) insists that his choice of goals is not normative: "The fact is that human physiologists have as yet found no functions clearly serving species survival rather than individual survival and reproduction." See also Boorse (2002, pp. 69, 76).

11. John A. Baker was helpful by highlighting this issue in correspondence.

12. This is not to say that we may never have legitimate reasons to count a grossly obese individual to be more "healthy" in comparison to another individual. However, I think such reasons will be essentially value-laden.

13. Some may object, though not in my view persuasively, against the contention that we must rely on, strictly speaking, human values. Consider that any legitimate appeal to an objective norm or value that is logically independent of human beings would seem to square off against Mackie's (1977) well-argued and forceful challenge to moral realism known as "the argument from queerness." I construe Mackie's attack to be against the thesis, roughly put, that claims there exist moral facts (or principles) and these moral facts (or principles) are logically independent of human beings.

14. Here, I also note the common standard of using a Bekker number to reference Aristotle: Nicomachean Ethics Book I: 1094b24–25. Interestingly, many of our contemporary views about health (e.g., the idea that health is a necessity for a flourishing life, the tendency to identify health narrowly in terms of bodily excellence, or much more widely with well-being) are to be found in the writings of Aristotle. See, for instance, Politics Book VII: 1330a38-b17 and Physics Book VII: 246b5. All references may be found in Aristotle (1984).

15. To illustrate, a search on the terms "definition," "concept," and "population health" in the databases Medline and Global Health would suggest that many writers simply presume there is no need to make explicit the account of health that underpins their particular research.

RESULTS OF SEARCHES ON POPULATION HEALTH, DEFINITION AND CONCEPT (DATE OF SEARCH: JULY. 30/10)			
SOURCE	TERM 1	TERM 2	RESULTS
	POP HEALTH		7828
MEDLINE	POP HEALTH	CONCEPT	182
	POP HEALTH	DEFINITION	89
	POP HEALTH		3328
GLOBAL HEALTH (OVID)	POP HEALTH	CONCEPT	59
	POP HEALTH	DEFINITION	45

16. I am grateful to Walter Glannon for valuable comments and suggestions on an earlier incarnation of this paper.

REFERENCES

Aristotle (trans., 1984). In J. Barnes (Ed.), *The complete works of Aristotle: The revised Oxford translation*. (Vols. 1–2). Princeton: Princeton University Press.

Boorse, C. (1975). On the distinction between disease and illness. *Philosophy and Public Affairs, 5*(1), 49–68.

Boorse, C. (1976). Wright on functions. *The Philosophical Review, 85*(1), 70–86.

Boorse, C. (1977). Health as a theoretical concept. *Philosophy of Science, 44*, 542–573.

Boorse, C. (1987). Concepts of health. In D. Van De Veer & T. Regan (Eds.), *Health care ethics: An introduction* (pp. 359–393). Philadelphia: Temple University Press.

Boorse, C. (1997). A rebuttal on health. In J. M. Humber & R. F. Almeder (Eds.), *What is disease?* (pp. 3–134). Towata, NJ: Humana Press.

Boorse, C. (2002). A rebuttal on functions. In A. Ariew (Ed.), *Functions: New essays in the philosophy of psychology and biology* (pp. 63–112). Oxford: Oxford University Press.

Canadian Public Health Association. (2008). *Canadian Public Health Association response to the World Health Organization (WHO) Commission's report*. Ottawa, ON.

Caplan, A. L. (1993). The concepts of health, illness and disease. In W.F. Bynum & R. Porter (Eds.), *Companion encyclopedia of the history of medicine, Vol. 1.* (pp. 233–248). London: Routledge.

Christensen, R. (2006). *Waterproof 2: Canada's drinking water report card*. Vancouver, B.C.: Sierra Legal Defence Fund.

Cooper, R. (2002). Disease. *Studies in History and Philosophy of Biological and Biomedical Sciences, 33* (2), 263–282.

Ereshefsky, M. (2009). Defining "health" and "disease." *Studies in the History and Philosophy of Biological and Biomedical Sciences, 40* (3), 221–227.

Frankish, C. J., Green, L. W., Ratner, P. A., Chomik, T. A., & Larsen, C. (1996). *Health impact assessment as a tool for population health promotion and public policy: A report submitted to the Health Promotion Development Division of Health Canada.* Vancouver, BC: University of British Columbia, Institute of Health Promotion Research.

Fulford, K.W.M. (1989). *Moral Theory and Medical Practice.* New York: Cambridge.

Kass, L. (1981). Regarding the end of medicine and the pursuit of health. In A. L. Caplan, H. T. Engelhardt, Jr., & J. J. McCartney (Eds.), *Concepts of health and disease: Interdisciplinary perspectives* (pp. 3–30). Reading, MA: Addison-Wesley.

Khushf, G. (1997). Why bioethics needs the philosophy of medicine: Some implications of reflection on concepts of health and disease. *Theoretical Medicine, 18,* 145–163.

Khushf, G. (2007). An agenda for future debate on concepts of health and disease. *Medicine, Health Care and Philosophy, 10,* 19–27.

Health Canada. (1998). *Taking action on population health: A position paper for Health Promotion and Programs Branch staff.* Ottawa, ON.

Health Canada. (2001). *The population health template: Key elements and actions that define a population health approach.* Ottawa, ON.

Nordenfelt, L. (1987). *On the nature of health: An action-theoretic approach.* Dordrecht: D. Reidel Publishing Company.

Nordenfelt, L. (2004). The logic of health concepts. In G. Khushf (Ed.), *The handbook of bioethics.* (pp. 205–222). Dordrecht: Kluwer Academic Publishers.

Mackie, J. L. (1977). *Ethics: Inventing right and wrong.* Harmondsworth, England: Penguin Books.

Mordacci, R., & Sobel, R. (1998). Health: A comprehensive concept. *Hastings Center Report, 28*(1), 34–37.

Pörn, I. (1993). Health and adaptedness. *Theoretical Medicine, 14*(4), 295–303.

PHAC (Public Health Agency of Canada). (2007). *Report on Plans and Priorities 2007–2008.*

PHAC (Public Health Agency of Canada). (2009). Website: http://www.phac-aspc.gc.ca/ph-sp/approach-approche/index-eng.php#def_health. Accessed December 1, 2009.

Reznek, L. (1987). *The Nature of disease.* London: Routledge and Kegan Paul.

Richman, K. A. (2004). *Ethics and the metaphysics of medicine.* Cambridge, MA: The MIT Press.

Senate of Canada (2008a). *Population health policy: Federal, provincial and territorial perspectives,* Third Report of the Senate Subcommittee on Population Health.

Senate of Canada (2008b). *Population health policy: Issues and options,* Fourth Report of the Senate Subcommittee on Population Health.

Stark, A. (2006). *The limits of medicine.* New York, NY: Cambridge University Press.

WHO (World Health Organization) (1946). *Constitution of the World Health Organization.* Official Records World Health Organization.

Towards an Ethical Framework for Population Health Research in Canada: A Place for Ethical Space?

Sylvia Abonyi, Shanthi Johnson, Diane Martz, Tom McIntosh, Nazeem Muhajarine, and Bonnie Jeffery

Health was described as "the ability to adapt to one's environment" by the French physician Georges Canguilhem in his 1943 essay *Le normal et le pathologique* (Canguilhem, 1978 English translation). If we apply this notion to the area of research, health research must be able to adapt to changing landscapes by learning from past practice and charting the course for future endeavours. This paper is concerned with trying to understand what the ethical dimensions of healthy population health research would look like, what we can learn from past practice, and how we can adapt to a changing environment.

While the study of population health is not new, past research practice has not translated into effective responses to the widely prevalent health disparities within and between countries. Nowhere is this truer than in the industrialized West, where despite support for and interest in population health research, and the immense productive capacity and wealth of those societies, they remain profoundly divided in terms of health outcomes between subpopulations. In addition to having limited positive impact on health disparities, population health research carries the risk of introducing negative impacts on vulnerable populations. Minimally, these include collecting data on issues when there is no guarantee that funding will be available to address them (Novins et al., 2004); and raising false hopes on the one hand, while painting a bleak health picture on the other hand (Lawn & Harvey, 2001).

Given the need to understand and address health disparities and the recent global resurgence of interest in addressing health disparities, most notably from the World Health Organization (WHO), we offered five recommendations for government action on health disparities via the social determinants of health that aim to balance local diversity with national coherence (Johnson et al., 2008). We include among these the argument that there is a need for promoting health equity by understanding the patterns, causes, and impacts of health disparities in populations and communities *through research that is community-engaged and policy-relevant*. This approach is foundational to a healthy population health research agenda that translates research into effective responses to ongoing global health disparities and at the same time minimizes potential negative impacts on vulnerable populations.

At its heart, healthy population health research must be rooted in a critical understanding of the ethical issues that emerge when confronting the health disparities of populations that, on a variety of fronts, are marginalized within dominant social, political, and economic structures. As Taylor and Johnson (2007) suggest, we must be concerned with the larger systemic effects that research in a particular population will have on that population. To understand what the ethical dimensions of healthy population health research look like, we begin by considering the ethical principles that currently guide population level research.

Pimple (2002), an ethicist, offers a series of questions for researchers to consider as they assess the ethics of their endeavour, questions that are useful to both individual- and population-level health research. He challenges us to ask: Is the research true? Is the research fair? Is the research wise? A "yes" answer to all three questions would suggest that the research is responsible and ethical. We will elaborate on these questions below, but begin with some important considerations that underpin our responses. As social scientists and population health researchers we would ground these questions in our belief that there are different ways of knowing and different approaches to knowledge that underscore the interdisciplinary and multi-stakeholder terrain of population health research and practice. While it would be possible to answer "yes" to all of Pimple's questions without taking these differences in approaches into account, we maintain that a healthy population health research agenda must find a way to accommodate them. To do otherwise would at best continue the status quo (limited translation of research into effective responses) or at worst continue to run the risk of unethical and potentially harmful research on the most vulnerable populations.

Foundational, therefore, to an affirmative response to Pimple's questions is that they take place in an ethical space that must include populations that are the focus of study (Ermine, 2000). The concept of ethical space is a process that both affirms the existence of different worldviews and knowledge systems and requires dialogue to act in a moral and ethical manner (Ermine, Sinclair, & Jeffery, 2004). It is in the ethical space that different knowledge systems engage and negotiate the research process through dialogue that will "encompass issues like language, distinct histories, knowledge traditions, values, interests, and social, economic and political realities and how these impact and influence an agreement to interact. Initially, it will require a protracted effort to create a level playing field where notions of hierarchy are replaced by concepts of equal relations" (Ermine, Sinclair, & Jeffery, 2004, p. 44). In this paper we consider Pimple's questions in turn as we grapple with a healthy population health research agenda that promotes health equity because it unfolds in an ethical space that is community-engaged and policy relevant.

IS IT TRUE?

With "truth" Pimple is referring to basic technical competence, the quality of data handling and manipulation, and the application of appropriate methodologies to arrive at the "truth." Population health researchers would do well to take a much broader approach to this question, calling into consideration "truth" at the level of conceptual development of our frameworks and measures. A central criticism of population health research is that it lacks a strong theoretical foundation (Frohlich, Corin, & Potvin, 2001; Weed, 2001; Williams, 2003; Carpiano & Daley, 2006). Rather, in an interdisciplinary enterprise, researchers in a range of fields bring with them concepts foundational to their disciplines and attempt to incorporate them under common interests in the health of populations.

The interdisciplinary dialogue, though rich and innovative, is accompanied by critiques that have ethical implications. Blalock (1990) captured these very well in a general critique of conceptual development and testing in social science research. He identifies some key "sins," all of which have ethical implications for arriving at "truth":

- *Applying theory and data at different levels of analysis.* Here Blalock considers the need to explicate the cross-level assumptions that are required whenever theories and the data used to test them are at different levels of analysis. He cautions that confusing and misleading interpretations may result when theoretical arguments pass between levels of explanation (for example, from individual to group or micro to macro) with little attention placed to the linkage between them and the level(s) of the data on which the argument rests. This is a classic challenge in population health where our theories about the impact of determinants on the health of populations play out at a collective level, yet the data we often work with is located at the level of the individual. Achieving collective level or systemic understandings requires aggregations that are based on cross-level assumptions that may or may not be fully considered.

- *Defining generic behaviour in such a way that either causes or effects are integral elements of the definition themselves.* Here Blalock is concerned with, for example, potentially oversimplifying assumptions behind the labels we assign behaviours. He offers the example of observations of "avoidance." We may assume (based on some theoretical or conceptual definition) that "avoidance" behaviour is motivated by the desire to reduce contact with some object, place, or person. If we then, for example, observe people moving away from one neighbourhood to another, do we then label that as "avoidance" according to our underlying assumption that moving away from something (defined as avoidance) is a desire to reduce contact with that something? Or might there be a multiplicity of other "motivators" for such a generic behaviour (for example, need for larger houses, increased employment proximity)?

- *Attempting precise but arbitrary measures where the reality being studied is inherently fuzzy.* Blalock considers this challenge with the example of how one might set about measuring "deviance" when the group norms upon which considerations of deviance might be based are themselves imprecise, ambiguous, and highly contextual. In terms of population health, a very good example can be drawn from our attempts to measure culture with precise measures (for example, participation in a certain activity) that may or may not represent a distinction between populations, where the differences in the norms that determine participation in that activity may be greater within population groups than between them.

- *Creating definitions based on convenience and data availability, rather than from theoretically derived criteria.* Population health researchers often access and attempt to link large regional, national, and international data sets that have been assembled for diverse purposes in different contexts driven by unspecified assumptions, none of which may be readily compatible with the empirical goals of a population health research question. As will be illustrated in the examples that follow, incompatibility in conceptualization at the measurement stage risks producing theoretically confusing interpretations or misinterpretations that may have little or negative impact on altering the health inequities that underpin a population health research agenda.

Carpiano and Daley (2006) comment on these "sins" specific to population health research, pointing out that "many of the models presented in population health research to date are discussed at such a high level of abstraction that their utility for constructing empirically testable hypotheses is stunted" (p. 565). Simply stated, the models are constructed at such an abstract level, and without showing pathways or linkages to lower levels of abstraction, that it is impossible to conceive of appropriate measures that would capture their intent. So a model that shows a broad link from culture to well-being without showing lower levels of abstraction that might theorize the mechanism creates a challenge in constructing a measure about culture that would capture the intent of the more abstract link. Another way to think of this is to look at the measures we use. We need to reflect on what determines our measures and whether they are actually measuring what we say they are measuring. In short, the assumptions underlying our indicators and measures must be reassessed. Koch (2000), for example, highlights the assumptions surrounding the concept of the quality of life. Specifically, he argues that the societal construction of the quality of life is narrow, based only on the burden of physical disease and disability supported by a medical model. Thus, the assumptions underlying these positions that relate to life quality ignore the very social, economic, and political conditions that provide the context for the construct. This is reflective of Blalock's concern about creating precise measures of realities that are, in actuality, quite fuzzy and imprecise. This practice is pervasive in national surveys and translates into how the measurement tools are constructed and subsequently used for gathering data.

Population health researchers commonly draw on large data sets, such as national surveys, that are collected for a variety of purposes not necessarily grounded in population health research concepts or frameworks, to address questions of importance to the health of populations. An additional ethical challenge to truth here is that the questions asked are often fraught with attitudes, values, and abilities *indirectly* inferred from the directly observed variables; assumptions that have not been explicitly and conceptually addressed. This is a case where Blalock might be concerned about the creation of definitions based on convenience and data availability, rather than conceptual rigour. For example, if we look at the gambling question in the Canadian Community Health Survey (Canada, 2009), we are asked:

In the past 12 months, how often have you bet or spent money on instant win/scratch tickets or daily lottery tickets (Keno, Pick 3, Encore, Banco, Extra)?

The interviewer is instructed to read the categories to the respondents and *exclude all other kinds of lottery tickets such as 6/49, Super 7, sports lotteries, and fundraising tickets.*

The exclusion of certain types of lottery tickets from the gambling questions raises questions about how we classify behaviours. This speaks directly to Blalock's concern for how behaviours are defined. For example, is it that gambling behaviour is reflected in the purchase of certain types of lottery tickets and not others? What are our assumptions about the motivations behind what we define as gambling behaviour? Are we assuming different motivations and, therefore, behaviour between the purchases of different kinds of tickets (how do we decide when it is gambling and when it is not)? Is it fair to measure gambling using a selective list? Is it wise to make the implication of acceptable and perhaps unacceptable types of gambling practices? Further, the response options appear to be arbitrarily set ("Daily," "Between 2 to 6 times a week," "About once a week," "Between 2 to 3 times a month," "About once a month," "Between 6 to 11 times a year," "Between 1 to 5 times a year," and "Never"). We need to explicitly ask what determines our choice of boundaries and what our assumptions are behind these boundaries. Is a judgment being made about those who buy a single Keno ticket every day relative to someone who buys a larger number of more expensive tickets once a week or once a month?

We also need to explicitly consider what determines which variables we group together and what our assumptions are behind these groupings. In another example, the National Population Health Survey (Canada, 1999) food security questionnaire assumes that the amount of money that people have available for food is affected by how much money they spend on housing. There may indeed be such a relationship, but the questions around this issue reflect a set of assumptions that may not, in fact, capture the relationship. The food security section of questions specifically asks, *"Do you or any other member of your household own this dwelling (even if it is still being paid for)?"* with the possibility of a "yes" or "no" response. This is followed by a question asking the respondents the amount of their regular mortgage payments. The assumption appears to be that mortgage payments are generally less than rental payments, thus freeing up money that can ensure greater food security. But mortgage payments are only one of the costs related to owning a home (for example, maintenance, property taxes, utilities, etc.) that may affect one's disposable income. In short, the assumptions built into the question may actually lead the researcher away from understanding the relationship between the cost of shelter and food security.

If we follow the example of survey tools a bit further, we must appreciate that the data and information we obtain is only as good as the questions asked and the response options provided. The nature of the questions asked and the way in which they are asked set and define the measures and parameters within which the participants are asked to respond. This can limit a wider array of potential responses and risks treating survey respondents as passive agents and creating demand characteristics, a psychological artefact in which the participants unconsciously change their responses to suit the researchers' objectives and expectations. From an ethical standpoint, the interplay between the assessor and the assessed is essential. Participants should be treated as active agents with a real and important stake in the research and with knowledge that may not correspond to the predetermined categories of the researcher. That is, involving participants and using an open-ended format overcomes the demand characteristics associated with a researcher-generated, structured format. Qualitative research instruments are equally as vulnerable to these challenges, where even an open-ended question can be quite misguided if it is the wrong question for a given context and not well-grounded conceptually (for example, asking someone where they live as opposed to where their home is might elicit very different responses for high-mobility versus low-mobility populations). Here we might fall into Blalock's trap of theorizing at one level and creating data at another, with unexplored assumptions about the nature of the linkage between the two. The solution here is not only to allow participants/subjects a role as active agents in responding—this is, after all, the norm for qualitative research—but to include the population from which they are drawn in setting the questions and interpreting the responses, as would be demanded of an ethical space approach.

The "truth" of population health research speaks to the way that various ideas and constructs are, first, defined or conceptualized and, second, the strength of the way these concepts are measured or operationalized either *qualitatively* or *quantitatively*. This "truth" should be viewed through an ethical lens, since the intent is to take findings directly to actions to reduce health inequities. Thus, the impacts of sloppy conceptualization and operationalization are hardly benign. At best, the impact of weakly conceptualized measures of population health on program or policy is absent (because no relationship between determinants and health can be empirically established). In such a case, the research fails at two levels. First, it fails its own test of being an accurate reflection of a reality shared by a population and, second, it fails to provide any real guidance regarding how health inequities might be reduced through social or political action. At worst, clumsy attempts to incorporate empirically weak or problematic associations between determinants and health can result in programs and policies that further marginalize the most vulnerable among us. Rather than reduce disparities between populations, such poorly designed interventions may indeed increase them. Tait (2007) offers a compelling discussion of these issues in the Canadian public health response to substance abuse by pregnant women in the "making" of fetal alcohol syndrome among Indigenous populations.

It is clear that there are challenges at the population level in answering "yes" to the first of Pimple's questions about ethical implications of research ("Is it true?"). We turn next to a discussion of fairness, which is every bit as challenging to consider at the level of populations.

IS IT FAIR?

In considering the fairness of research, Pimple would have us consider the nature of the relationship between participants/subjects and researchers. Ethical guidelines for the protection of individual human subjects are not new in the health research arena. There are internationally recognized ethical guidelines for research with human subjects, with roots in the Nuremberg Code (1947), the Declaration of Helsinki (1964), the Belmont Report (1979), and the Universal Declaration of Bioethics and Human Rights (2005).[1] Canada has adopted eight principles enshrined in these documents in the Tri-Council Policy Statement (TCPS), which guides researchers at colleges and universities who receive funding from the three national research funding agencies which make up the Tri-Council: Canadian Institutes of Health Research (CIHR), Natural Sciences and Engineering Research Council of Canada (NSERC), and Social Sciences and Humanities Research Council of Canada (SSHRC).[2] Researchers are required to adhere to these principles with evidence of protocols receiving ethical approval from institutional research ethics boards (REBs). The Canadian principles include:

- Respect for human dignity;
- Respect for free and informed consent;
- Respect for vulnerable persons;
- Respect for privacy and confidentiality;
- Respect for justice and inclusiveness;
- Balancing harms and benefits; and
- Non-maleficence and beneficence. (CIHR, NSERC & SSHRC, 1998, pp. i.5-i.6)

Ironically, while they were developed in response to moral and ethical violations against vulnerable populations, all of these early guidelines and principles are focused on the protection of the individual. Protection of populations, therefore, is limited to an aggregation of individual protections that assumes an autonomous decision-maker free of contingencies and contexts

(Wallwork, 2002). In one sense, this is not surprising, given the dominant Western positivist research paradigm that seeks to aggregate and disaggregate information to control for some factors while revealing objective and universal truths about another. However, as Wallwork (2002) argues, an individualistic approach effectively cuts individuals off from the histories, relationships, and communities in which they are embedded. In addition, Taylor and Johnson (2007) correctly point out that population-based measures affect all members of a particular group, regardless of one individual's choice to participate or not. There is, therefore, a need also to consider ethical protections at the level of populations.

Although the most recent draft second edition of the Tri-Council policy statement in Canada focuses on only three core principles, for the first time the interplay of individuals and the groups of which they are part is explicitly recognized in these three principles.

The first core principle is welfare, which encompasses not only the well-being of individuals, but also, more broadly, the individual's physical, social, economic, and cultural environments. The discussion around this principle recognizes that research can impact not only the individual, but also those communities of which the individual is part. Recognizing that the benefits of population level research may accrue over a long timeline, while the risks assumed by a population may be more immediate (for example, stigma), Taylor and Johnson (2007) add that we should ask: "How much *potential* societal benefit must be possible, to counter-balance such risks?" (p. 298).

The second core principle is autonomy and refers to free and informed consent. This principle also has implications beyond the individual, as the document states that

> the exercise of autonomy is influenced by an individual's various connections: to family; to community; and to cultural, social, linguistic, religious and other groups.... and that under some conditions, the views of the groups affected may have to be considered by the researcher and the REB in approving the research. (Interagency Advisory Panel on Research Ethics, 2008)

The third core principle of respect for the equal moral status of all humans speaks to the requirement that the benefits and burdens of research must be distributed equally and that particular groups should not be discriminated against. Past research abuses have led to the recognition that some groups in society need extra protection. However, a delicate balance exists when affording vulnerable groups extra protection, while ensuring those groups are not denied access to participation in ethical research that, in the area of population health research, could reduce the inequities that produce their particular sets of vulnerabilities (Interagency Advisory Panel on Research Ethics, 2008).

The diverse nature of the collectives of interest to population health research adds a further challenge in applying our current ethical principles (as is being reflected in the new draft second edition TCPS), and in constructing a population health research ethics framework. Some groups may be more highly structured and bounded, such as on-reserve First Nations groups, and others may be linked by a very few shared interests, such as urban neighbourhoods. Wallwork (2002) challenges us to consider a number of questions related to intra-group diversity: When does a group become worthy of a separate collective ethic? How should harms and benefits be weighed if there are contradictions between the interests of individuals versus the group? Who represents the group?

As with the question "is it true?" the question "is it fair?" puts specific demands on the population health researcher, demands that have not always been met in practice. It requires a very conscious and conspicuous critical reflection on the part of the researcher both before and during the research process. And it requires us to appreciate—if not fully comprehend—the perspectives of those with whom we conduct research. Pondering the fairness of the research should push us further in our engagement in a dialogue with those populations with whom we work, and speaks again to the requirement that we open up the research process from the outset to create an ethical space that includes "the subject" as a true "participant" in the research. It is, after all, the participants' communities that the research should be designed to serve.

IS IT WISE?

In many ways this is one of the most difficult and important of Pimple's questions to address for population health research. For Pimple, the wisdom of the research speaks to its contribution to the common good and to its fiscal responsibility. The population research enterprise by definition is about common good and ascribes to values of social justice (Taylor & Johnson, 2007). For population health, achieving wisdom in research is about finding a way forward through the dilemmas we are presented with under "truth" and "fairness." Given the range of disciplines and stakeholders involved, notions of "truth" and "fairness" play out on a field of competing agendas and interests. The way forward, as others have already identified (Carpiano & Daley, 2006), is to adopt a perspective that accepts that there are different knowledge systems at play in the population health research and practice agendas. From this standpoint, then, one is forced to accept that there are multiple truths that can be revealed through the greater involvement by the populations of focus—and the recognition and inclusion of the lay knowledge they possess—in the research enterprise (Taylor & Johnson, 2007). Fairness is achieved through a reconciliation of differences that respects and protects the validity of each stakeholder's knowledge system. Here, some precedent exists and is embodied in the CIHR *Guidelines for Ethical Research with Aboriginal Peoples* (CIHR, 2007). In the document, ethicist Willie Ermine argues for the notion of an ethical space, wherein the reconciliation of differences is possible. For research with Canadian Aboriginal populations, this translates into the application of the principles of ownership, control, access, and possession (OCAP) (Schnarch, 2004). Researchers, in partnership with Aboriginal stakeholders, negotiate questions regarding the ownership, control, access, and possession of research projects, data, and dissemination, which are ideally located in the population/community context. For the larger population health research enterprise, the practical translation, at minimum, means a participatory process that includes the early involvement by stakeholders in collectively

- determining and resourcing research priorities;
- creating conceptual frameworks that accommodate different knowledge systems;
- applying appropriate measurement and analytical tools;
- interpreting findings; and
- determining outcomes.

There are some good examples of the success of this approach in Canada (see, for example, Abonyi & Jeffery, 2006; Ball & Janyst, 2008; Jacklin & Kinoshameg, 2008; Martens & Fransoo, 2008; Muhajarine et al., 2007; Thompson et al., 2007; O'Neil & Blanchard, 2001). These ideas are not, however, confined within the borders of Canada. In a series of papers sponsored by the National Institutes of Health (NIH) in the United States, authors specifically consider where and how community-driven processes have helped address problems regarding research ethics and the social responsibility of the researcher (see, for example, Wing, 2001; Quigley, 2001). Let us turn again to the example of measurement to see what this would mean. While it is true that Canada has excellent data on individual and population health indicators through national and provincial surveys, such as the Canadian Community Health Survey discussed above, we can go part of the way to addressing some of the issues around truth and fairness identified earlier with a coordinated and integrated population health information infrastructure that includes culturally appropriate, community-relevant indicators identified with community and population stakeholders (Johnson et al., 2008). Further, data and information from national surveys are powerful tools in understanding and addressing health disparities, but they only assess traditional quantitative indicators such as life expectancy, mortality, and morbidity. Thinking ethically from a population health perspective, researchers ought to be reflecting, with appropriate stakeholders, if these indicators truly reflect the health of individuals and communities. Lalonde (2005, p. 21) offers an approach in which we could ask four basic questions:

- What is a healthy community?
- How would we measure that?
- How healthy is our community?
- Why would we measure that?

The last question is reflective, allowing us to revisit and revise our answers to the first three. Even for measures that are valid and conceptually sound, we still need to consider the underlying values associated with the choice and use of these traditional indicators and their relevance for various communities. Is it fair to equate health of populations to the level of disability or morbidity? Is it wise to continue to use only these indicators that do not take into account the social and cultural contexts? There is a need and an opportunity to include other indicators relevant to various communities (Jeffery et al., 2006). While quantitative indicators are beneficial, integration of qualitative research and evidence is needed—and desired—to add depth and nuance in the understanding and the addressing of health disparities.

CONCLUSION

At minimum, for the development of a healthy population health research framework, we should be guided by Pimple's questions about responsible and ethical research, bearing in mind the many nuances discussed in this paper. Traditional positivist science and social science would insist that only the objective scientist could answer Pimple's three questions and, indeed, would allow that scientist to define the conditions under which the answer to any or all of them would be "yes."

However, if researchers take seriously the existence of multiple kinds of knowledge, mulitple systems of knowledge, and multiple ways of knowing, then they must look to methods and frameworks that allow those multiplicities to be brought forward. Dialogue between researchers and populations can open up an ethical space where the two can share those different ways of knowing and, ultimately, where the answers to the questions "is it true?" "is it fair?" and "is it wise?" are negotiated as partners in a shared enterprise that blurs the distinction between researcher and researched. In attempting to answer Pimple's three questions from within that ethical space, we are challenging ourselves to conduct our research in profoundly different ways and with, we hope, a greater likelihood that its outcomes will have greater meaning, importance, and impact for those whose health inequities are the greatest.

NOTES

1. See Mitscherlich & Mielke (1949) for the Nuremberg Code; see World Medical Association (1964) for the Declaration of Helsinki; see National Commission for the Protection of Human Subjects of Biomedical and Behavioral Research (1979) for the Belmont Report; see UNESCO (2005) for the Universal Declaration of Bioethics and Human Rights.
2. The agencies of the Tri-Council are funded by the federal government and award grants on the basis of peer-reviewed competition. There are also a number of provincial research funding agencies that operate in a similar manner.

REFERENCES

Abonyi, S., & Jeffery, B. (2006). Evaluative tools for community-based Aboriginal health organizations. Case study. *Moving population and public health knowledge into action. A casebook of knowledge translation stories.* CIHR-CIHI.

Ball, J., & Janyst, P. (2008). Enacting research ethics in partnership with Indigenous communities in Canada: "Do it in a good way." *Journal of Empirical Research on Human Research Ethics, 3*(2), 33–51.

Blalock, H. M. (1990). Auxiliary measurement theories revisited. In J. J. DeLong-Gierveld & J. Hox (Eds.), *Operationalization and research strategy* (pp. 33–48). Amsterdam: Stets and Zeitlinger.

Canguilhem, Georges. (1978). *On the normal and pathological,* trans. Carolyn R. Fawcett. Dordrecht, Holland: D. Reidel.

Carpiano, R. M., & Daley, D. M. (2006). A guide and glossary on post-positivist theory building for population health. *Journal of Epidemiology and Community Health, 60,* 564–570.

Canada. Statistics Canada. (1999). National Population Health Survey. Retrieved from http://www.statcan.gc.ca/concepts/nphs-ensp/index-eng.htm

Canada. Statistics Canada. (2009). *Canadian Community Health Survey.* Retrieved from http://www.statcan.gc.ca/concepts/health-sante/content-contenu-eng.htm

CIHR (Canadian Insitutes of Health Research). (2007). CIHR *guidelines for health research involving Aboriginal peoples.* Ottawa: CIHR.

CIHR, NSERC & SSHRC (Canadian Institutes of Health Research, Natural Sciences and Engineering Research Council of Canada, Social Sciences and Humanities Research Council of Canada). (1998 [with 2000, 2002 and 2005 amendments]). *Tri-council policy statement: Ethical conduct for research involving humans.* Accessed December 7, 2009. http://pre.ethics.gc.ca/eng/policy-politique/tcps-eptc/

Ermine, W. J. (2000). The ethics of research involving Indigenous peoples. Unpublished Master's thesis, University of Saskatchewan.

Ermine, W.J., Sinclair, R., & Jeffery, B. (2004). The ethics of involving Indigenous peoples: A report of the Indigenous Peoples Health Research Centre to the Interagency Advisory Panel on Research Ethics. Saskatoon, SK: Indigenous Peoples Health Research Centre. Retrieved December 7, 2009. http://www.iphrc.ca/IPHRCResearchdocs.php.

Frohlich, K., Corin, E., & Potvin, L. (2001). A theoretical proposal for the relationship between context and disease. Sociology of Health and Illness, 23(6), 776–797.

Interagency Advisory Panel on Research Ethics. (2008). Draft Second edition of the Tri-council policy statement: Ethical conduct for research involving humans. Interagency Secretariat on Research Ethics. Retrieved December 7, 2009. http://pre.ethics.gc.ca/eng-/policy-politique/initiatives/draft-preliminaire/

Jacklin, K., & Kinoshameg, P. (2008). Developing a participatory Aboriginal health research project: "only if it is going to mean something." Journal of Empirical Research on Human Research Ethics, 3(2), 53–68.

Jeffery, B., Abonyi, S., Labonte, R., & Duncan, K. (2006). Engaging numbers: Developing health indicators that matter for First Nations and Inuit people. Journal of Aboriginal Health, 3(1), 44–52.

Johnson, S., Abonyi, S., Jeffery, B., Hackett, P., Hampton, M., McIntosh, T., Martz, D., Muhajarine, N., Petrucka, P., & Sari, N. (2008). Recommendations for action on the social determinants of health: A Canadian perspective. The Lancet, 372, 1690–1693.

Koch, T. (2000). Life quality vs the 'quality of life': Assumptions underlying prospective quality of life instruments in health care planning. Social Science & Medicine, 51, 419–427.

Lalonde, C. (2005). Creating an index of healthy Aboriginal communities. In Developing a healthy communities index: A collection of papers. Ottawa: Canadian Institute of Health Information.

Lawn, J., & Harvey, D. (2001). Change in nutrition and food security in two Inuit communities, 1992–1997. Report prepared for Indian and Northern Affairs Canada, Ottawa.

Martens, P., Fransoo, R. et al. (2008). What works? A first look at evaluating Manitoba's regional health programs and policies at the population level. Winnipeg: Manitoba Centre for Health Policy.

Mitscherlich, A., & Mielke, F. (Eds.). (1949). The Nuremberg Code [1947]. In Doctors of infamy: The story of the Nazi medical crimes (pp. xxiii-xxv). New York: Schuman.

Muhajarine, N., Glacken, J., Cammer, A., & Green, K. (2007). KidsFirst Program evaluation-Phase 1. Evaluation framework. University of Regina and University of Saskatchewan: Saskatchewan Population Health and Evaluation Research Unit.

National Commission for the Protection of Human Subjects of Biomedical and Behavioral Research. (1979). The Belmont report: Ethical principles and guidelines for the protection of human subjects of research. Department of Health, Education, and Welfare. Retrieved December 7, 2009. http://www.hhs.gov/ohrp/humansubjects/guidance/belmont.htm.

Novins, D. K., LeMaster, P. L., Jumper Thurman, P., & Plested, B. (2004). Describing community needs: Examples from the Circles of Care initiative. American Indian and Alaska Native Mental Health Research, 11(2), 42–58.

O'Neil, J. D., & Blanchard, J. (2001). Considerations for the development of public health surveillance in First Nations communities. Assembly of First Nations: Health Secretariat and First Nations Information Governance Committee, Ottawa.

Pimple, K. D. (2002). Six domains of research ethics: A heuristic framework for the responsible conduct of research. Science and Engineering Ethics, 8, 191–205.

Quigley, D. (2001). Research ethics issues with Native American communities. In D. Quigley (Ed.), Compilation on environmental health research ethics issues with Native communities. Unpublished manuscript funded by a grant from the National Institutes of Health, National Institute of Allergies and Infectious Disease Grant Program for Research Ethics-T15A149650–01.

Schnarch, B. (2004). Ownership, control, access and possession (OCAP), or self-determination applied to research: A critical analysis of contemporary First Nations research and some options for First Nations communities. *Journal of Aboriginal Health, 1*(1), 80–95.

Tait, C. (2007). Disruptions in nature, disruptions in society: Indigenous peoples of Canada and the "making" of Fetal Alcohol Syndrome. In L. Kirmayer & G. Valaskakis (Eds.), *The mental health of Canadian Aboriginal peoples: Transformations of identity and community.* Vancouver: University of British Columbia Press.

Taylor, H. A., & Johnson, S. (2007). Ethics of population-based research. *The Journal of Law, Medicine, and Ethics, 35*(2), 295–299.

Thompson, L., Shand, S., Jeffery B., McIntosh, T., Abonyi, S., & Martz, D. (2007). *Phase 1. Evaluation frameworks for the Aboriginal health human resources initiative and the Aboriginal health transition fund.* Regina & Saskatoon: Saskatchewan Population Health and Evaluation Research Unit.

UNESCO. (2005). Universal Declaration on Bioethics and Human Rights. Retrieved December 7, 2009. http://unesdoc.unesco.org/images/0014/001461/146180E.pdf.

Wallwork, E. (2002). Ethical analysis of group and community rights: Case study review of the "Collaborative initiative for research ethics in environmental health." In Dianne Quigley (Ed.), Compilation on environmental health research ethics issues with Native communities. Unpublished manuscript funded by a grant from the National Institutes of Health, National Institute of Allergies and Infectious Disease Grant Program for Research Ethics-T15A149650–01.

Weed, D. L. (2001). Theory and practice in epidemiology. *Annals of the New York Academy of Science, 954,* 52–62.

Williams, G. H. (2003). The determinants of health: Structure, context and agency. *Sociology of Health and Illness, 25,* 131–154.

Wing, S. (2001). Social responsibility and research ethics in community driven studies of industrialized hog production. In Dianne Quigley (Ed.), Compilation on environmental health research ethics issues with Native communities. Unpublished manuscript funded by a grant from the National Institutes of Health, National Institute of Allergies and Infectious Disease Grant Program for Research Ethics-T15A149650–01.

World Medical Association. (1964 [with amendments 1975, 1983, 1989, 1996, 2000, 2002, 2004, 2008]). *Declaration of Helsinki.* Accessed December 7, 2009. http://www.wma.net/en/30publications/10policies/b3/index.html

Income Inequality and Health: A Theoretical Quagmire

Nadine Nowatzki

INTRODUCTION

Over a hundred years ago, Durkheim (1897/1966) observed that people who were socially isolated were more likely to commit suicide. More recently, research on the social determinants of health has expanded to address the relationships between a number of socio-economic predictors and health outcomes. Health sociologists and social epidemiologists now understand that sickness and death are not random, but rather occur in distinct patterns that are socially produced. A plethora of studies has examined the relationship between socio-economic status and health, demonstrating that regardless of how health outcomes are measured, individuals with lower levels of income, education, and occupational status experience poorer health and earlier death (Ross et al., 2006).

However, the relationship between socio-economic status (SES) and health involves more than just poverty. Classic studies of hierarchies and health (see Marmot et al., 1991; Townsend & Davidson, 1982) revealed a social "gradient" in health representing the relationship between low-to-high SES and the correlated high-to-low risk for morbidity and mortality (Wermuth, 2003). Studies of SES and health have proliferated, confirming that each step up the gradient is associated with better health outcomes than the rung below. This means that it is not only the poor who are affected by the gradient: even among the middle and upper classes, those with lower relative rankings suffer more disease and earlier death than those with higher rankings (Daniels, Kennedy, & Kawachi, 2000; Lynch & Kaplan, 2000; Raphael, 2004). Researchers also observed that several governments invest in social programs and have good health and literacy outcomes in spite of considerable poverty. For example,

Costa Rica and Cuba have more relative equality, despite low gross domestic product and relatively low average incomes (Coburn, 2004; Sen, 1999).

As a result of these observations, as well as trends of increasing inequality in wealthy nations since the 1970s, the past 15 years have witnessed a new focus in academic research on the health effects of the *relative* distribution of income in a society. Some researchers have argued that the degree of inequality in a society, rather than the absolute level of poverty or an individual's own income, is more important in affecting health (e.g., Wilkinson, 2006). Income inequality is therefore a characteristic of a group or place (aggregate level), rather than an individual attribute such as income.

Several review papers (e.g., Wilkinson & Pickett, 2006) have examined the growing body of literature on income inequality and health, highlighting in particular the methodological considerations. However, comparatively less attention has been paid to the role of theory. The purpose of my paper is to focus on the theoretical issues surrounding the income inequality hypothesis. I will begin by providing a brief review of the income inequality and health literature. Next, I will discuss two proposed pathways through which income inequality is hypothesized to affect health. These two frameworks— *psychosocial* and *neo-material*—have dominated the literature. I will then outline other theoretical orientations that have received much less attention. These include the *political economy, cultural-structuralist, social exclusion,* and *intersectional* frameworks. I will highlight the potential contributions of these frameworks to understanding the causal linkages between social inequality and health disparities. The paper concludes with a discussion of the research and policy implications of more theoretically grounded research.

INCOME INEQUALITY AND HEALTH: A BRIEF REVIEW OF THE LITERATURE

Cross-national research examining the link between income inequality and health spans several decades, but intensified in the early 1990s with the publication of Wilkinson's (1992) analyses. He reported a strong correlation between income inequality and life expectancy, and concluded that it is the distribution of income rather than the absolute wealth of a country that is strongly related to health differences between countries—the greater the gap between the rich and the poor, the worse the health outcomes for the population (Wilkinson, 1992, 1996, 2006).

A detailed examination of the income inequality literature is not possible for the purposes of this paper. In short, although several subsequent cross-national studies found strong associations between income inequality and health outcomes in developed countries (e.g., Duleep, 1995; Wennemo, 1993), some researchers have critiqued Wilkinson's data and analyses (e.g., Judge, 1995; Judge, Mulligan, & Benzeval, 1998), while others have failed to replicate or support his findings (e.g., Beckfield, 2004; Lynch et al., 2001). State-level studies, and investigations conducted in metropolitan areas, census tracts, and counties, have also had mixed results, with some researchers finding support for the income inequality hypothesis (e.g., Lynch et al., 1998; Ram, 2005). On the other hand, other researchers have reported more modest associations, associations limited to particular age groups or incomes, or evidence of confounding variables, such as racial composition or education, that account for the observed relationship between income inequality and health (e.g., Deaton & Lubotsky, 2003; Mellor & Milyo, 2002, 2003).

Review articles have pointed to these inconsistent findings as well as the methodological limitations of research to date, concluding that the relationship between income inequality and health is unclear (see Lynch et al., 2004; Macinko et al., 2003; Subramanian & Kawachi, 2004; Wagstaff & van Doorslaer, 2000). Limitations include the use of cross-sectional data, rather than longitudinal and prospective data; the use of different models in each study; the lack of multi-level studies; inconsistent measures/indicators of income inequality and health outcomes; inclusion of different control variables; different data and time periods; small samples; and different combinations of countries or states. These limitations make it difficult to compare studies, and even when the same data and outcome measures have been used, there have been contradictory findings. The strongest evidence for the effects of income inequality on health are among U.S. states, but even that evidence is somewhat mixed. At this point in time, it is not possible to make any definitive conclusions about the relationship between income inequality and health (Lynch et al., 2004).

EXPLAINING INEQUALITY AND HEALTH: PSYCHOSOCIAL AND NEO-MATERIAL FRAMEWORKS

In the mid- to late 1990s, the vast majority of published studies supported the income inequality hypothesis, and researchers began to outline the pathways through which income inequality might affect health. Although the relationship between income inequality and health is far from clear, it is still important to explore and understand the frameworks that have guided much of the research on the income inequality hypothesis. Two frameworks in particular have generated considerable debate.

Psychosocial Explanations
Several researchers belong to what is referred to as the "neo-Durkheimian" (Muntaner & Lynch, 1999) tradition and hypothesize that psychosocial

mechanisms explain the health effects of inequality. Wilkinson (1996, 1999) was one of the earliest proponents of a psychosocial explanation. He has emphasized relative poverty and the processes of stressful social comparisons, suggesting that people interpret their place in the social hierarchy by comparing their social circumstances to those of other people. Poor health is believed to result from these processes of invidious social comparison. A widening gap between the rich and poor results in relative deprivation, including: feelings of shame, stress, anxiety, frustration, lower self-esteem, distrust, and loss of control. These result in poor health outcomes due to psycho-neuro-endocrine mechanisms, that is, the mind-body connection (Kawachi & Kennedy, 1997; Wilkinson, 1996, 1999).

Poor health outcomes may also stem from unhealthy lifestyle behaviours that low-income individuals use to cope. Current public policy continues to focus on health behaviours (e.g., diet, exercise) as an explanation for health inequalities. However, this "blame-the-victim" approach fails to recognize that lifestyle behaviours are strongly correlated with SES, with lower income groups less likely to engage in health-protective behaviours. The high cost of healthier foods and recreational activities obviously plays a role, as does the ability to "buy" time (e.g., child care, housekeeping) to take advantage of such resources. However, health-threatening behaviours such as smoking and substance use are also responses to deprivation, uncertainty, and powerlessness, and thus have a psychosocial stimulus (Raphael, 2004, 2007).

The psychosocial approach may overstate the role of social comparisons, and the explanations that have been offered for how social hierarchy affects health have been largely intuitive and simplistic. Research on reference groups is sparse, and there is little consensus on how or with whom people compare their situation (Kawachi, 2000). A Scottish study found that "social comparisons of homes," that is, perceiving one's home or apartment to be inferior to those around one, was related to poorer psychosocial health (Ellaway et al., 2004). It is not known if social comparisons of homes would be related to poorer *physical* health, and it is important to note that social comparisons of cars was not significantly related to poorer psychosocial health.

The majority of income inequality studies utilizing a psychosocial framework have focused on "social capital." Most writers have included these terms under the psychosocial umbrella, referring to them as the "macro-level" version of the psychosocial framework (e.g., Lynch & Kaplan, 1997; Lynch et al., 2000; Macinko et al., 2003; Macinko, Shi, & Starfield, 2004). According to this version, income disparities damage the social fabric within societies, resulting in a breakdown of social bonds. A widening gap between the rich and the poor leads to a marked increase in residential segregation and the spatial concentration of poverty and affluence. Social cohesion is undermined due to a disinvestment in social capital, indicated by low levels of trust, low levels of involvement in voluntary organizations, and low voter turnout (Kawachi & Kennedy, 1997, 1999, 2002).

Social capital is viewed as a community asset with features such as civic participation and engagement, norms of reciprocity, trust in others, confidence in government, social cohesion, and values of cooperation, tolerance, and solidarity (Coleman, 1988; Putnam, 1993, 1995). Studies of the relationship between inequality, social capital, and health have had mixed results, with some researchers finding support for the social capital pathway (e.g., Kawachi et al., 1997) and others finding weak and inconsistent associations (e.g., Lynch et al., 2001).

The social capital framework has stirred up controversy and criticism. In particular, the framework lacks a plausible explanation of why social capital is important to health (Wilkinson, 1999), and "plausibility is a rather weak criterion for establishing causality" (Macleod & Davey Smith, 2003, p. 565). Several writers have criticized the methodologies used in social capital research, arguing that the empirical association with health is unclear and is by no means causal (Muntaner, Lynch, & Davey Smith, 2001; Pearce & Davey Smith, 2003). Macleod and Davey Smith (2003) suggest that the relationship between psychosocial factors and physical disease may reflect reverse causation (due to the use of cross-sectional research designs), reporting bias, and especially, residual confounding by unmeasured aspects of the material environment that are typically related to stress and other psychosocial factors.

Islam et al. (2006) note that there are ambiguities concerning whether social capital is an individual or collective attribute. There is no shared definition of what social capital and social cohesion are or do, or how to achieve them (Labonte, 2004). The definitions have been notoriously inconsistent, vague, shallow, tautological, and difficult to operationalize, yet they have been adopted and applied uncritically (Lynch et al., 2000b; Muntaner & Lynch, 1999; Portes, 1998). In some cases, social capital is merely a labelling of previously used concepts such as social support (Portes, 1998).

The social capital approach has also been criticized for romanticizing communities by assuming homogeneity and shared interests and by downplaying struggle and conflict. Politics, class relations, exploitation, and power have been ignored in most social capital research (Muntaner & Lynch, 1999; Muntaner, Lynch, & Davey Smith, 2001; Navarro, 2002). While social networks can be a source of social support, they can also be coercive and function as a source of strain. One group's social capital (e.g., the Mafia) can be another group's oppression (Lynch et al., 2000a, 2000b; Portes, 1998). Social cohesion can undermine autonomy if a community or social group demands conformity, excludes others, or restricts freedoms; and social support that is negative in quality can be detrimental to health (Islam et al., 2006; Macinko & Starfield, 2001).

Kubzansky and Kawachi (2000) maintain that research on emotions and health could lead to "the development of psychosocial interventions which aim to break the link between social conditions and illness outcomes" (p. 231). However, critics argue that targeting individuals or communities to increase their levels of social capital may "blame the victim," create resentment, and be ineffective or even harmful (Pearce & Davey Smith, 2003). Macleod and Davey Smith (2003) are skeptical that "counseling poor people to 'cheer up' or 'relax' or 'take more control' without changing their access to material resources will improve their physical health" (p. 568). It is important to note, however, that most social capital researchers do not advocate for psychosocial interventions targeting unhealthy feelings, but rather focus on more upstream policies and programs. In addition, a focus on psychosocial dynamics does not necessarily mean that material or structural factors are unimportant.

Nevertheless, psychosocial measures that are more proximal to health are susceptible to being decontextualized and depoliticized. Traditional epidemiological measures of SES and social capital, often stemming from Durkheimian theory, tend to be individually specified, reductionistic, and understood within a vacuum. Such measures may fail to capture the more distal macro-level structural determinants, including social, legal, and economic policies, and their effects on the distribution of individual characteristics across the population (Lynch & Kaplan, 2000; Pearce & Davey Smith, 2003). Lynch et al. (2000a) argue that the political-economic processes that produce inequality exist *prior* to people's perceptions of inequality and hence their experiences of social cohesion.

Measures of social capital clearly need further theoretical grounding, conceptual clarity, and psychometric testing to determine their validity and reliability and to allow comparability between studies (Macinko & Starfield, 2001). Otherwise, it is difficult to understand how the various manifestations of the social capital concept "could be linked" to the specific risk factors for particular population health outcomes and how these change over time" (Davey Smith & Lynch, 2004, p. 700).

Neo-materialist Explanations
Drawing on both Marxist and Weberian traditions, Lynch and Kaplan (1997, 2000) propose a neo-materialist approach to understanding the relationship between inequality and health. They attribute health differences to the

control of economic, material, political, and cultural resources, which are differentially distributed within a population. As a result of social and political processes, those who are exploited in capitalist societies face more negative exposures and demands, but tend to have the least access to, or control over, resources that might buffer their disproportionate levels of stress. Structural processes therefore generate different opportunities or "life chances."

Lynch and Kaplan (1997) note that "income distribution is a characteristic of a social system" (p. 298), and they argue that the focus should be on the properties of the social and economic systems in which people live. Obviously, individual characteristics and behaviours are important in determining health outcomes; however, an understanding of health behaviours and outcomes must recognize the socio-political context in which they take place. Policies that affect wages, investments, and taxes are important determinants of income inequality and, hence, individual outcomes (Lynch et al., 2000a).

According to Lynch and Kaplan (1997), "inequitable income distribution may be associated with a set of social processes and policies that systematically underinvest in human, physical, health and social infrastructure, and this underinvestment may have health consequences" (p. 306). Neo-materialists argue that jurisdictions where high income inequality is tolerated are less likely to provide equitable resources such as education, housing, or environmental protection. Higher levels of social expenditures, as well as strategic social investments and redistributive actions, are viewed as the route to more equality and better health. Some evidence for this proposed pathway comes from a study on state inequality and mortality in the United States. The states with more equitable income distribution spent more on social infrastructure and had better health outcomes (Kaplan et al., 1996).

The neo-materialist approach has been criticized for being too diffuse, seeming to embrace "everything but the genome" (Marmot & Wilkinson, 2001, p. 1234). Some have suggested that in wealthier nations, basic material needs (e.g., heat, water, electricity) are met and it cannot be argued that they directly affect health behaviour (Wilkinson & Pickett, 2006). Critics further argue that ensuring the provision of certain material goods as well as a safe and healthy environment will not eliminate health disparities, as hierarchies and their psychosocial implications will continue to affect health. In particular, a gradient occurs even among those who are not poor, suggesting the importance of psychosocial factors (Marmot & Bobak, 2000).

Neo-material advocates, however, "do not deny that social inequality has psychosocial costs for individuals, or that these negative psychosocial effects are an important topic for public health" (Lynch et al., 2000b, p. 406). Nevertheless, a focus on perceptions of relative income can direct attention away from differences in real income, especially at the low end of the income distribution where the greatest burden of poor health exists (Lynch et al., 2000b). Even in wealthier countries, there are populations lacking basic material necessities, as evidenced by the living conditions on some Canadian First Nations reserves. Interestingly, a Swedish study found that the health effects of relative deprivation disappeared at low-income levels, suggesting that absolute income was more important to health for the 40 percent with the lowest incomes (Yngwe et al., 2003). Even amongst higher income grades, where basic material needs for housing and food are met, there is likely to be differential access to neo-material aspects of life that may include quality child care, education, health care, neighbourhoods, and recreation. These resources are important determinants of health and well-being (Lynch et al., 2000b).

THE ROADS LESS TRAVELLED:
OTHER POTENTIAL EXPLANATORY FRAMEWORKS

The debate between psychosocial and neo-material writers has dominated the literature on income inequality and health, with researchers from each camp critiquing the other's approach. Unfortunately, this has ultimately served to narrow the scope of focus by distracting attention from other potential directions for investigation. There are numerous potential explanatory frameworks that merit exploration, yet they have received relatively little attention. In this section, I will discuss four of these approaches.

Political Economy

Political economy is a structural perspective that also stems from the work of Marx, particularly his analysis of exploitation within capitalist systems. Within a political economy approach, "States, markets, ideas, discourses, and civil society are not independent variables but interrelated parts of the same whole" (Armstrong, Armstrong, & Coburn, 2001, p. vii). This perspective focuses on the causes of inequality, rather than only on the health consequences of inequality. This includes the production, reproduction, and persistence of inequalities (Coburn, 2000, 2004; Muntaner & Lynch, 1999; Scambler, 2002). A political economy approach is congruent with a neo-materialist approach, but has a broader view. For example, it highlights how global political and economic forces, such as trade agreements, structure social life (Wermuth, 2003).

From a political economy approach, health is also viewed in the context of class relations and ruling. In particular, the roles of ideology and power are examined (Raphael, 2004; Scambler, 2002). Several political economists note that the welfare state in many developed countries has been weakened through economic globalization and the adoption of neo-liberal approaches that emphasize the role of markets in determining the allocation of resources. The neo-liberal mantra is decidedly anti-statist and advocates liberalization (free markets, free trade), privatization, deregulation, and a reduced role for the welfare state. According to neo-liberal ideology, the hardships of the poor are necessary costs in order to accelerate economic development (Coburn, 2000, 2004; Labonte, 2004).

States have different responses to the pressures of corporations and globalization depending on the dominant ideology and welfare state type and the power of corporate interests. Policy is therefore influenced by the political climate. Welfare states with the least state action and the most dominant market-oriented solutions, such as the United States and Canada, have seen rapid and dramatic increases in inequality, greater poverty, and increasing health disparities compared to the more collectivist Nordic countries. Theorists such as Coburn (2000, 2004) argue that neo-liberalism is responsible for both increased inequality and lowered social cohesion, and both result in poorer health outcomes. Thus, progressive welfare state policies that include redistribution are important both in material terms and in psychosocial terms.

There is a growing body of evidence that illustrates the relationship between welfare state policies and health outcomes. Cross-national comparisons have shown that higher levels of taxation and social spending are associated with better health outcomes (Davey Smith, 1996; Kaplan et al., 1996; Lynch et al., 2000a). Several studies have found that the political ideologies of governing parties in wealthy countries affect population health. Political traditions with egalitarian ideologies (e.g., social democratic parties in the Nordic countries) tend to implement universalistic and redistributive policies aimed at reducing social inequalities. These policies seem to be more successful at improving population health (Navarro et al., 2006; Navarro & Shi, 2001).

There are very few studies in the income inequality and health literature that have employed a political economy perspective, and, as a result, there have been few critiques of its explanatory power. On the positive side, this literature moves our focus from individual bodies and behaviours to the social structural context as the locus of a population's health (Weber & Parra-Medina, 2003).

However, as with the psychosocial and neo-material approaches, there is a tendency to equate social class with income, which is a very limited variable. Thus, most researchers conceptualize income and wealth as vertical or distributional constructions of inequality (having more), rather than horizontal or relational constructions (having power over) (Veenstra, 2007; Weber & Parra-Medina, 2003). Moreover, a primary focus on income inequality means that other measures, such as race and sex, are treated as "add-ons." This is a limited approach given that health inequalities result from the clustering of disadvantage within specific historical and cultural contexts (Raphael, 2001).

To address these limitations, broader and more complex theoretical approaches are needed. Recent work using the concept of *social exclusion*, Bourdieu's *cultural-structuralist* framework, and feminist *intersectional* approaches hold a great deal of promise for capturing and making visible these relational constructions.

Social Exclusion

The term social exclusion refers to the multi-dimensional societal processes that contribute to certain groups (e.g., women, Aboriginals, visible minorities) being systematically denied the opportunity to participate in society (Raphael, 2007). Social exclusion is viewed as both a process and an outcome that includes not only isolation, but also exclusion from political participation and decision-making, as well as social and cultural activities (Galabuzi, 2004). Social exclusion denies people access to important social goods such as decent housing, education and training, and transportation, due to racism, discrimination, hostility, and unemployment (Wilkinson & Marmot, 2003).

Rather than focusing solely on poverty (a "distributional" concept), social exclusion draws attention to the multi-dimensional, dynamic, relational, and spatial aspects of deprivation and disadvantage (Room, 1999). Labonte (2004) proposes that the term "social exclusion" is more sophisticated and useful because it directs attention to the social structuring of relationships and the role of political systems and power in affecting health. This approach expands our focus beyond excluded groups and their conditions, to address excluding (capitalist) structures, that is, the socio-economic ideologies and policies that exclude groups and create unequal conditions. This "upstream" version of social exclusion overlaps with neo-materialist and political economy approaches. It has the potential to bridge the divide between the various perspectives because it allows for an understanding of the relationships between material disadvantage, excessive psychosocial stress caused by uncertainty and lack of control, and unhealthy behaviours, and the resulting health outcomes (Raphael, 2001; Wilkinson & Marmot, 2003).

Despite its apparent potential, a social exclusion framework has yet to be employed in income inequality and health studies, and instead seems to be aimed at replacing studies of poverty (income) and health. And although the framework appears to have numerous advantages, a number of issues will need to be addressed before it can be used fruitfully as an explanatory framework. Like social capital, it is a notoriously difficult concept to define, let alone measure. At times it seems to be used synonymously with poverty, social capital, or social cohesion approaches. In addition, despite the promise to focus on excluding structures, much of social exclusion research to date has continued to focus on "the excluded," which draws the focus away from the political processes that contribute to exclusion. In this sense, it is a "softer" term than poverty, diverting attention away from massive inequalities and potentially leading to the pathologization of excluded groups. Much of the social exclusion work has tended to propose insertion or integration strategies without questioning the fundamental organization of society that results in exclusion in the first place (Bowring, 2000; Levitas, 2005; Raphael, 2007; Ratcliffe, 1999).

Cultural-structuralist

Recently, several health writers (e.g., Abel, 2008) have adopted Bourdieu's cultural-structuralist approach to understand the health effects of inequality. This relational framework expands beyond the economic realm and defines classes in social space by their possession and use of various resources or "capitals." The concept of social space refers to groupings of similarly located individuals who may share circumstances and potentially be social classes. Whereas some writers have interpreted social space as an actual physical or geographical space, such as neighbourhood networks (e.g., Carpiano, 2006), Veenstra (2007) focuses on the social and psychological aspects of the social space. These include cultural tastes and dispositions, as well as lifestyle practices, which dominant groups may use to "maintain boundaries between themselves and lesser groups by delineating the nature of tastes—legitimate, middle-class, and popular, or high-brow, middle-brow and low-brow—and then utilizing familiarity with these cultural forms to exclude others" (p. 16). In his exploratory study, Veenstra used multiple correspondence analysis (MCA) to examine the relations between categories of variables. He found that educational and economic capital were the defining dimensions of social space and that positions in social space were related to differences in self-rated health and depression.

The use of Bourdieu's concept of social capital is relatively recent and has not been utilized to a great extent within the income inequality and health literature. However, some limitations have surfaced. For example, social capital may be related more with mental health than with physical health (Ziersch et al., 2005). It has also been argued that the exclusive focus on geographical location is not a fruitful one, particularly since neighbourhood cannot be equated with community, and social spaces can be dispersed across geographical space (Gatrell et al., 2004; Stephens, 2008). Such a communitarian approach to Bourdieu's concepts of capital fails to recognize the importance of the wider social and political context. Access to, and competition over, various capitals was central to Bourdieu's theory of practice (Stephens, 2008).

Bourdieu's network-based theory and concepts of capital do have the potential to shift our attention from the poor to the role of the wealthy in working to maintain status and resources, and perpetuating inequalities by excluding others from health-promoting resources (Stephens, 2008). Although health research has relied heavily on Putman's conceptualization of social capital, some have argued that Bourdieu's concept holds far greater theoretical promise (e.g., Portes, 1998).

Intersectionality

An intersectional approach developed through the interdisciplinary and post-colonial theorizing of feminists from developing countries and European/American feminists of colour. The purpose of an intersectional analysis is "to explicate the socially constructed and intricately intertwined nature of race, class, gender, and sexuality systems of inequality" (Weber & Parra-Medina, 2003, p. 184). Conceptual and analytical knowledge of such intersectionalities is needed to understand and respond to the multiple effects of interlocking inequalities on health (Schulz & Mullings, 2005). This approach would acknowledge and make visible the complex and dynamic interface between simultaneous inequalities, allowing us to explore how dimensions of difference interconnect and mutually reinforce each other (Hankivsky, 2005; Weber & Parra-Medina, 2003). This draws attention to broader hierarchies, as well as the specific historical and cultural contexts that contribute to injustice. There is great potential for significantly expanding, complicating, and deepening our knowledge of health inequalities (Weber & Parra-Medina, 2003; Whittle & Inhorn, 2001).

Some writers have cautioned, however, that intersectionality is conceptually, theoretically, and methodologically "murky," and has rarely been applied empirically (Nash, 2008). Definitions of intersectionality are vague, and although it can be a useful analytical tool, it needs to be theoretically differentiated to understand how the intersections of various categories of difference interact with the lived experience of subjects (Staunæs, 2003). Several writers also note that due to the complexity of including multiple categories of analysis, multiple and unique methodological approaches are needed. Yet there is a lack of defined methodologies for studying intersectionality, and the empirical validity of intersectionality remains problematic. There has been a great deal of discussion surrounding *why* we should study intersectionality, but little discussion of *how* to study it. The failure to overcome disciplinary boundaries has meant that little mainstream work is being done to develop and embrace multiple approaches to the study of intersectionality (McCall, 2005).

Viewed from social exclusion, cultural-structuralist, or intersectional perspectives, an exclusive focus on income or wealth as isolated and independent inequalities is clearly inadequate and limits our approaches to eliminating health inequalities (Hankivsky, 2005; Weber & Parra-Medina, 2003; Whittle & Inhorn, 2001). It will be interesting to see how future studies of income inequality and health are able to broaden their perspective utilizing these more comprehensive frameworks.

CONCLUSION

It would seem that we need "many windows on the world," and that each of these explanations of the relationship between inequality and health offers us valuable insight and potential avenues for action. Scambler (2002) doubts that there are "discrete and identifiable 'pathways'" between class relations, social cohesion, inequality, and health. Rather, "there are likely to be innumerable, different and changing routes to the same end points" (p. 104). It should not be surprising that research has found evidence to support both material and psychosocial aspects of inequality (e.g., Pikhart et al., 2003). Researchers from opposing camps agree that some of the explanatory frameworks are linked, with both material and psychosocial pathways between inequality and health (Lynch & Kaplan, 1997; Wilkinson & Marmot, 2003). For example, Pearce and Davey Smith (2003) argue that material and political factors are major determinants of both social capital and health inequalities. Thus, psychosocial factors play a role, but are just one of several potential pathways between macro-level forces and health.

It is clear that the various approaches are not contradictory, but are rather complementary and, in some cases, overlapping. Most of these explanations point to the role of broader social structures in determining the level of inequality in a society. An understanding of the psychosocial pathways between income inequality and health is also valuable, provided we look beyond these more proximal determinants of health and recognize that such pathways are "inextricably linked to the material features of the environment" (Lynch & Kaplan, 1997, p. 308; Muntaner, Lynch, & Davey Smith, 2001). Sociological and social epidemiological approaches that include a neo-materialist and political economy approach are necessary in order to understand the causes of inequality on a broader global scale and the processes through which social stratification is reproduced, rather than only the health consequences of inequality (Lynch & Kaplan, 2000; Scambler, 2002).

Szreter and Woolcock (2004) have proposed a comprehensive framework that attempts to reconcile the psychosocial, material, and political economy perspectives into a coherent social capital theory. In addition to previously theorized "bonding" and "bridging" forms of social capital, they propose a "linking" form that occurs between people who are interacting across power or authority gradients in society. Although interesting, very few researchers have explored these concepts or applied the framework. However, the framework has already drawn sharp criticism for continuing to ignore the social and political mechanisms and power relations (class, race, and gender relations) that generate inequalities in the first place (e.g., Muntaner, 2004).

Despite the debates over the pathways between income inequality and health, one comment is consistently made in this literature: the importance of theory in guiding research and the need for future researchers to conduct further theoretical work (Carpiano & Daley, 2006). This requires researchers to move beyond the divisive psychosocial versus neo-material debate to more productive theory building and operationalization. Comprehensive conceptual and theoretical frameworks can help to address both substantive and methodological issues surrounding the income inequality hypothesis, including the issue of adjustment for confounding (Kawachi & Kennedy, 1999; Lynch & Kaplan, 1997). Such frameworks also permit the use of appropriately complex and theoretically grounded statistical methods such as confirmatory factor analysis and structural equation modelling. Researchers need to specify health models that link their theoretical and empirical hypotheses, and test competing pathways. The choice of indicators should also be justified on theoretical grounds (Macinko et al., 2003).

Interestingly, Raphael et al. (2005) analyzed 241 Canadian studies of income and health, and found that fewer than half had offered explicitly structural theorizations. Furthermore, close to a third did not explicate *any* pathways mediating the relationship between income or income distribution and health. They argue that more interdisciplinary work could contribute to more sophisticated conceptualizations of the pathways. The predominance of biomedical and epidemiological approaches to health, which view health in an individualistic, superficial, and decontextualized manner, may be part of the problem. For example, Muntaner, Lynch, and Davey Smith (2001) argue that the concept of social capital employed in the public health literature lacks depth compared with its uses in the social sciences. More contributions from social scientists, including sociologists and political scientists, would likely shed light on the processes through which income and its distribution affect health (Raphael et al., 2006). Health research informed by social science conceptualizations has a greater potential to highlight political and economic processes and point to upstream policy implications.

In conclusion, although a causal relationship between income inequality and health has not been unequivocally supported, it remains a very important research area with potentially crucial policy implications. In Canada, there is growing inequality of income and especially wealth, yet we are witnessing a deteriorating public policy environment focused more on lifestyle and bio-medical frameworks than on structural determinants of health (Raphael et al., 2005, 2006). If evidence supporting a relationship between income inequality and health were firmer, the argument for redistributive policies would be much stronger. Reducing inequality by redistributing resources to the most disadvantaged will improve the health of the poor and increase average population health (Lynch et al., 2004; Subramanian & Kawachi, 2004). Unfortunately, current research approaches rarely publish policy implications that address the distribution of social and economic resources among the population. Suggestions that a society change how it distributes such resources remain controversial (Raphael et al., 2005).

REFERENCES

Abel, T. (2008). Cultural capital and social inequality in health. *Journal of Epidemiology & Community Health, 62*(7), e13.

Armstrong, P., Armstrong, H., & Coburn, D. (Eds.). (2001). *Unhealthy times: Political economy perspectives on health and care.* Don Mills: Oxford University Press.

Beckfield, J. (2004). Does income inequality harm health? *Journal of Health & Social Behavior, 45,* 231–248.

Bowring, F. (2000). Social exclusion: Limitations of the debate. *Critical Social Policy, 20*(3), 307–330.

Carpiano, R. M. (2006). Toward a neighborhood resource-based theory of social capital for health: Can Bourdieu and sociology help? *Social Science & Medicine, 62,* 165–175.

Carpiano, R. M., & Daley, D. M. (2006). A guide and glossary on post-positivist theory-building for population health. *Journal of Epidemiology & Community Health, 60,* 564–570.

Coburn, D. (2000). Income inequality, lowered social cohesion, and the poorer health status of populations: The role of neo-liberalism. *Social Science & Medicine, 51,* 135–146.

Coburn, D. (2004). Health, health care, and neo-liberalism. In Armstrong, P., H. Armstrong, & D. Coburn (Eds.), *Unhealthy times: Political economy perspectives on health and care in Canada* (pp. 45–65). Don Mills, ON: Oxford University Press.

Coleman, J. (1990). *The foundations of social theory.* Cambridge, MA: Harvard University Press.

Daniels, N., Kennedy, B., & Kawachi, I. (2000). *Is inequality bad for our health?* Boston: Beacon Press.

Davey Smith, G. (1996). Income inequality and mortality: Why are they related? *British Medical Journal, 312,* 987–989.

Davey Smith, G., & Lynch, J. (2004). Social capital, social epidemiology and disease aetiology. *International Journal of Epidemiology, 33*(4), 691–700.

Deaton, A., & Lubotsky, D. (2003). Mortality, inequality and race in American cities and states. *Social Science & Medicine, 56,* 1139–1153.

Duleep, H. O. (1995). Mortality and income inequality among economically developed countries. *Social Security Bulletin, 58,* 34–50.

Durkheim, E. (1897/1966). *Suicide.* New York: Free Press.

Ellaway, A., McKay, L., Macintyre, S., Kearns, A., & Hiscock, R. (2004). Are social comparisons of homes and cars related to psychosocial health? *International Journal of Epidemiology, 33,* 1065–1071.

Galabuzi, G. E. (2004). Social exclusion. In D. Raphael (Ed.), *Social determinants of health: Canadian perspectives* (pp. 235–252). Toronto: Canadian Scholars' Press Inc.

Gatrell, A., Popay, P., & Thomas, C. (2004). Mapping the determinants of health inequalities in social space: Can Bourdieu help us? *Health & Place, 10,* 245–257.

Hankivsky, O. (2005). Gender vs. diversity mainstreaming: A preliminary examination of the role and transformative potential of feminist theory. *Canadian Journal of Political Science, 38,* 977–1001.

Islam, M. K., Merlo, J., Kawachi, I., Lindstrom, M., & Gerdtham, U. G. (2006). Social capital and health: Does egalitarianism matter? A literature review. *International Journal for Equity in Health, 5,* 3–63.

Judge, K. (1995). Income distribution and life expectancy: A critical appraisal. *British Medical Journal, 311,* 1282–1285.

Judge, K., Mulligan, J., & Benzeval, M. (1998). Income inequality and population health. *Social Science & Medicine, 46,* 567–579.

Kaplan, G., Pamuk, E., Lynch, J., Cohen, R., & Balfour, J. (1996). Inequality in income and mortality in the United States: Analysis of mortality and potential pathways. *British Medical Journal, 312,* 999–1003.

Kawachi, I. (2000). Income inequality and health. In L. Berkman and I. Kawachi (Eds.), *Social epidemiology* (pp. 76–94). New York: Oxford University Press.

Kawachi, I., & Kennedy, B. P. (1997). Health and social cohesion: Why care about income inequality? *British Medical Journal, 314,* 1037–1045.

Kawachi, I., & Kennedy, B. P. (1999). Income inequality and health: Pathways and mechanisms. *Health Services Research, 34,* 215–226.

Kawachi, I., & Kennedy, B. P. (2002). *The health of nations: Why inequality is harmful to your health.* New York: New Press.

Kawachi, I., Kennedy, B. P., Lochner, K., & Prothrow-Stith, D. (1997). Social capital, income inequality, and mortality. *American Journal of Public Health, 87,* 1491- 1498.

Kubzansky, L. D., & Kawachi, I. (2000). Affective states and health. In L. F. Berkman & I. Kawachi (Eds.), *Social epidemiology* (pp. 213–241). New York: Oxford University Press.

Labonte, R. (2004). Social inclusion/exclusion and health: Dancing the dialectic. In D. Raphael (Ed.), *Social determinants of health: Canadian perspectives* (pp. 253–266). Toronto: Canadian Scholars' Press Inc.

Levitas, R. (2005). *The inclusive society? Social exclusion and new labour* (2nd ed.). Basingstoke: MacMillan.

Link, B., & Phelan, J. (1995). Social conditions as fundamental causes of disease. *Journal of Health & Social Behavior, Spec,* 80–94.

Lynch, J., Davey Smith, G., Harper, S., Hillemeier, M., Ross, N., Kaplan, G.A., & Wolfson, M. (2004). Is income inequality a determinant of population health? Part I. A systematic review. *Milbank Quarterly, 82*(1), 5–99.

Lynch, J., Davey Smith, G., Hillemeier, M., Shaw, M., Raghunathan, T., & Kaplan, G. (2001). Income inequality, the psychosocial environment, and health: Comparisons of wealthy nations. *The Lancet, 358,* 194–200.

Lynch, J., Davey Smith, G., Kaplan, G., & House, J. (2000a). Income inequality and mortality: Importance to health of individual income, psychosocial environment, or material conditions. *British Medical Journal, 320,* 1220–1224.

Lynch, J., Due, P., Muntaner, C., & Davey Smith, G. (2000b). Social capital: Is it a good investment strategy for public health? *Journal of Epidemiology & Community Health, 54,* 404–408.

Lynch, J. W., & Kaplan, G. A. (1997). Understanding how inequality in the distribution of income affects health. *Journal of Health Psychology, 2*(3), 297–314.

Lynch, J. W., & Kaplan, G. A. (2000). Socioeconomic position. In L. Berkman and I. Kawachi (Eds.), *Social epidemiology* (pp. 13–35). New York: Oxford University Press.

Lynch, J., Kaplan, G., Pamuk, E., Cohen, R., Balfour, J., & Yen, I. (1998). Income inequality and mortality in metropolitan areas of the United States. *American Journal of Public Health, 88,* 1074–1080.

Macinko, J. A., Shi, L., & Starfield, B. (2004). Wage inequality, the health system, and infant mortality in wealthy industrialized countries, 1970–1996. *Social Science & Medicine, 58,* 279–292.

Macinko, J. A., Shi, L., Starfield, B., & Wulu, J. (2003). Income inequality and health: A critical review of the literature. *Medical Care Research & Review, 60*(4), 407–452.

Macinko, J., & Starfield, B. (2001). The utility of social capital in research on health determinants. *The Milbank Quarterly, 79,* 387–427.

Macleod, J., & Davey Smith, G. (2003). Psychosocial factors and public health: A suitable case for treatment? *Journal of Epidemiology & Community Health, 57,* 565–570.

Marmot, M., & Bobak, M. (2000). International comparators and poverty and health in Europe. *British Medical Journal, 321,* 1124–1128.

Marmot, M., Davey Smith, G., Stansfeld, D., Patel, D., North, F., et al. (1991). Health inequalities among British civil servants: The Whitehall II study. *Lancet, 337,* 1387–1392.

Marmot, M., & Wilkinson, R.G. (2001). Psychosocial and material pathways in the relation between income and health: A response to Lynch et al. *British Medical Journal, 322,* 1233–1236.

McCall, L. (2005). The complexity of intersectionality. *Signs: Journal of Women in Culture and Society, 30,* 1771–1800.

Mellor, J. M., & Milyo, J. (2003). Is exposure to income inequality a public health concern? Lagged effects of income inequality on individual and population health. *Health Services Research, 38,* 137–151.

Mellor, J. M., & Milyo, J. (2002). Income inequality and individual health: Evidence from the Current Population Survey. *Journal of Human Resources, 37,* 510–539.

Muntaner, C. (2004). Social capital, social class, and the slow progress of psychosocial epidemiology. *International Journal of Epidemiology, 33,* 674–680.

Muntaner, C., & Lynch, J. (1999). Income inequality, social cohesion, and class relations: A critique of Wilkinson's Neo-Durkheimian research program. *International Journal of Health Services, 29,* 59–81.

Muntaner, C., Lynch, J., & Davey Smith, G. (2001). Social capital, disorganized communities, and the Third Way: Understanding the retreat from structural inequalities in epidemiology and public health. *International Journal of Health Services, 31,* 213–237.

Nash, J. C. (2008). Re-thinking intersectionality. *Feminist Review, 89*, 1–15.

Navarro, V. (2002). A critique of social capital. *International Journal of Health Services, 32,* 423–432.

Navarro, V., Muntaner, C., Borrell, C., Benach, J., Quiroga, A., Rodriguez-Sanz, M., Verges, N., & Pasarin, M. (2006). Politics and health outcomes. *The Lancet, 368*(9540), 1033–1037.

Navarro, V., & Shi, L. (2001). The political context of social inequalities and health. *Social Science & Medicine, 52,* 481–491.

Pearce, N., & Davey Smith, G. (2003). Is social capital the key to inequalities in health? *American Journal of Public Health, 93,* 122–129.

Pikhart, H., Bobak, M., Rose, R., & Marmot, M. (2003). Household item ownership and self-rated health: Material and psychosocial explanations. *BMC Public Health, 3,* 38–44.

Portes, A. (1998). Social capital: Its origins and applications in modern sociology. *Annual Review of Sociology, 24*(1), 1–24.

Putnam, R. (1993). *Making democracy work: Civic traditions in modern Italy.* Princeton, NJ: Princeton University Press.

Putnam, R. (1995). Bowling alone: America's declining social capital. *Journal of Democracy, 6,* 65–78.

Ram, R. (2005). Income inequality, poverty, and population health: Evidence from recent data from the United States. *Social Science & Medicine, 61,* 2568–2576.

Raphael, D. (2001). *Inequality is bad for our hearts: Why low income and social exclusion are major causes of heart disease in Canada.* Toronto: North York Heart Health Network.

Raphael, D. (2004). Introduction to the social determinants of health. In D. Raphael (Ed.), *Social determinants of health: Canadian perspectives* (pp. 1–18). Toronto: Canadian Scholars' Press Inc.

Raphael, D. (2007). *Poverty and policy in Canada: Implications for health and quality of life.* Toronto: CPSI.

Raphael, D., Labonte, R., Colman, R., Hayward, K., Torgerson, R., & MacDonald, J. (2006). Income and health in Canada: Research gaps and future opportunities. *Canadian Journal of Public Health, 97,* S16-S23.

Raphael, D., MacDonald, J., Colman, R., Labonte, R., Hayward, K., & Torgerson, R. (2005). Researching income and income distribution as determinants of health in Canada: Gaps between theoretical knowledge, research practice, and policy implementation. *Health Policy, 72,* 217–232.

Ratcliffe, P. (1999). Housing inequality and "race": Some critical reflections on the concept of "social exclusion." *Ethnic & Racial Studies, 22,* 1–22.

Room, G. J. (1999). Social exclusion, solidarity and the challenge of globalization. *International Journal of Social Welfare, 8*(3), 166–174.

Ross, N., Wolfson, M., Kaplan, G. A., Dunn, J. R., Lynch, J., & Sanmartin, C. (2006). Income inequality as a determinant of health. In J. Heymann, C. Hertzman, M. L. Barer, and R. G. Evans (Eds.), *Healthier societies: From analysis to action* (pp. 202–236). New York: Oxford University Press.

Scambler, G. (2002). *Health and social change: A critical theory.* Philadelphia, PA: Open University Press.

Schulz, A. J., & Mullings, L. (Eds.). (2005). *Gender, race, class and health: Intersectional approaches.* San Francisco: Jossey-Bass.

Sen, A. (1999). *Development as freedom.* New York: Oxford University Press.

Staunæs, D. (2003). Where have all the subjects gone? Bringing together the concepts of intersectionality and subjectification. *NORA: Nordic Journal of Women's Studies, 11*(2), 101–110.

Stephens, C. (2008). Social capital in its place: Using social theory to understand social capital and inequalities in health. *Social Science & Medicine, 66,* 1174–1184.

Subramanian, S. V., & Kawachi, I. (2004). Income inequality and health: What have we learned so far? *Epidemiologic Reviews, 26,* 78–91.

Szreter, S., & Woolcock, M. (2004). Health by association? Social capital, social theory, and the political economy of public health. *International Journal of Epidemiology, 33,* 650–667.

Townsend, P., & Davidson, N. (1982). *Inequalities in health: The Black report.* Harmondsworth, England: Penguin.

Veenstra, G. (2007). Social space, social class and Bourdieu: Health inequalities in British Columbia, Canada. *Health & Place, 13,* 14–31.

Wagstaff, A., & van Doorslaer, E. (2000). Income inequality and health: What does the literature tell us? *Annual Review of Public Health, 21,* 543–567.

Weber, L., & Parra-Medina, D. (2003). Intersectionality and women's health: Charting a path to eliminating health disparities. In M.T. Segal, V. Demos, & J. Jacobs Kronenfeld (Eds.), *Gender perspectives in health and medicine: Key themes* (pp. 181–230). Oxford: Elsevier.

Wennemo, I. (1993). Infant mortality, public policy and inequality: A comparison of 18 industrialized countries 1950–1985. *Sociology of Health & Illness, 15,* 429–446.

Wermuth, L. (2003). *Global inequality and human needs: Health and illness in an increasingly unequal world.* Boston: Allyn and Bacon.

Whittle, K. L., & Inhorn, M. C. (2001). Rethinking difference: A feminist reframing of gender/race/class for the improvement of women's health research. *International Journal of Health Services, 31*(1), 147–165.

Wilkinson, R. G. (1992). Income distribution and life expectancy. *British Medical Journal, 304,* 165–168.

Wilkinson, R. G. (1996). *Unhealthy societies: The afflictions of inequality.* New York: Routledge.

Wilkinson, R. G. (1999). Health, hierarchy, and social anxiety. *Annals of the New York Academy of Sciences, 896,* 48–63.

Wilkinson, R. G. (2006). *The impact of inequality: How to make sick societies healthier.* New York: The New Press.

Wilkinson, R., & Marmot, M. (Eds.). (2003). *Social determinants of health: The solid facts* (2nd ed.). Copenhagen, Denmark: World Health Organization.

Wilkinson, R. G., & Pickett, K. E. (2006). Income inequality and population health: A review and explanation of the evidence. *Social Science & Medicine, 62,* 1768–1784.

Yngwe, M. A., Fritzell, J., Lundber, O., Diderichsen, F., & Burstrom, B. (2003). Exploring relative deprivation: Is social comparison a mechanism in the relation between income and health? *Social Science & Medicine, 57,* 1463–1473.

Ziersch, A. M., Baum, F. E., MacDougall, C., & Putland, C. (2005). Neighbourhood life and social capital: The implications for health. *Social Science & Medicine, 60,* 71–86.

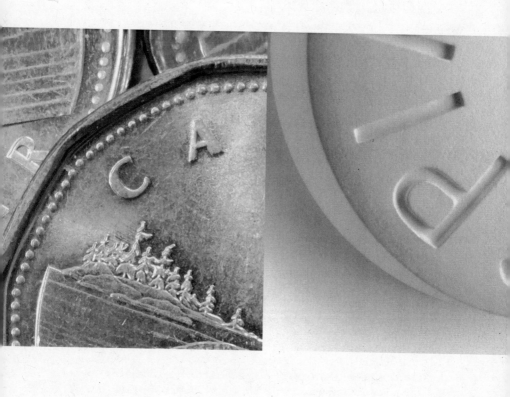

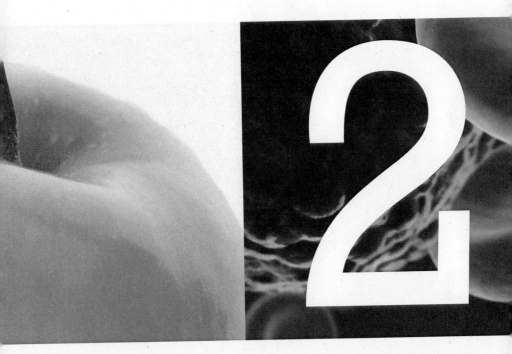

CRITICAL POPULATION HEALTH

Aboriginal Health Research and Epidemiology: Differences between Indigenous and Western Knowledge

Ulrich Teucher

According to epidemiological evidence, and many newspaper reports, we know that "by almost every measure, Aboriginal people are sicker and die younger than other Canadians" (Sallot 2004, p. A5). They die from conditions that include inordinately high rates of (among other things) birth defects, infant death, diabetes, and suicide. The numbers for Aboriginal youth suicide are particularly alarming. Native young persons take their own lives at a rate that is not only many times higher than that of other Canadians (five to seven times the national average; Health Canada, 2006), but at rates higher than for any culturally identifiable group in the world (Kirmayer, 1994). What we need to know is how it is possible that such an extreme health disparity could have come to pass in Canada and how it can be eradicated.

In our own decade-long search for answers to the problem of Aboriginal youth suicide we have found that suicide rates are indeed dramatic when calculated across the whole of Canada's diverse Aboriginal populations. However, we have also found that these numbers do not fairly describe the life and death circumstances facing any particular Aboriginal community. For example, in British Columbia, where our own research has been conducted, 90 percent of all Aboriginal youth suicides occur in only 10 percent of the bands. Some bands suffer youth suicide rates several hundred times the national average, while over half of the province's bands have not experienced a single youth suicide in the 13-year period for which figures are now available (Chandler, Lalonde, Sokol, & Hallett, 2003).

It is a tragic event when even a single young person commits suicide. In this regard it may matter little whether a suicide is counted as evidence of a national trend or as an individual occasion in a local context. But where this does matter, and matters importantly, is with regard to the scope of the policies that we may decide upon in order to improve existing health disparities. General epidemiological calculations of Aboriginal youth suicide rates across Canada can further beliefs that these problems are part of an assumed "Aboriginal condition"; that Canada's Aboriginal peoples cannot take care of themselves; and that government must intervene. By contrast, accounting for apparent differences in youth suicide rates between individual bands demonstrates that many bands are not faced with a suicide problem; can indeed take care of themselves; and possess real knowledge that produces rearing environments in which young people find life worth living. Evidently, some Aboriginal communities either lack this knowledge, or are somehow unable to bring it into practice (Chandler, Lalonde, & Teucher, 2003). What is apparent, then, is that traditional, top-down transfers of government health knowledge have not worked. If, instead, local bands could be enticed to share their existing knowledge "laterally" with each other, those bands that are doing less well could perhaps benefit. However, so far, several impediments seem to have limited such sharing, including the ignorance of researchers and government regarding differences between Indigenous and Western knowledge, cultural differences between Aboriginal peoples, and notions of the place-specificity of Indigenous knowledge with regard to "the land." Acknowledging these differences may lead to new directions for epidemiologists as we gather data and must decide to what extent this knowledge may or may not be generalizable, and what conclusions and policies we might formulate with regard to knowledge transfers of "best practices."

The balance of this chapter is about how such "knowledge transfers" might be facilitated, and, more specifically, about finding ways around those impediments that threaten to block the effective "exchange" of such best practices. What requires being said on this topic falls roughly into three parts. Part one concerns differences between Western and Indigenous knowledge systems as an explanation for some of the reasons why government bureaucracies and the academy have failed to acknowledge the possibility that real solutions to important social problems, such as youth suicide, might already be present within the larger Aboriginal community itself. Part two addresses some of the potential obstacles to the shareability of Indigenous knowledge, in particular with regard to the strong ties to the "land" found in Aboriginal knowledge systems, and aims to work out how ways might be found around such obstacles. Part three provides a summary of our ongoing research into youth suicide, exemplifying the need in Aboriginal health research to conduct epidemiological studies at the level of individual bands.

PART ONE: WHOSE KNOWLEDGE, WHOSE BEST PRACTICES?

The questions regarding what is to count as knowledge, and how such knowledge is best shared, arise everywhere there is a need to know. Until quite recently, much of Western thought believed that knowledge, and the thought processes that form knowledge, are a universal feature, to be perfected through universally applicable logic and scientific practices. However, recent research has been suggesting that there are different ways of thinking in the world. In his book, *The Geography of Thought: How Asians and Westerners Think Differently*, Richard Nisbett (2003) points out that much of Western thinking and its understanding of science originated in the classical Greeks' conceptualizations of nature as a collection of discrete and independent parts, that is, as an object of study to be categorized by human minds. In contrast, Chinese philosophers are said to have viewed the world as a matrix of interdependent interactions in which parts could only be understood in their interrelations with the whole (Nisbett, 2003, pp. 18–19). These different attitudes are said to have resulted in disparate epistemic postures, famously, those reared in "individualistic" versus "collectivist" cultures (Hofstede, 1980; Markus & Kitayama, 1991; Triandis, 1995; Nisbett, Peng, Choi, & Norenzayan, 2001). Some philosophers of language have gone even further, suggesting that it is not so much social or cultural differences, but the various structures of our languages that are differently constitutive of the ways we think about ourselves and the world, thereby shaping differences in epistemologies. Related and equally general claims have been made by various scholars of Aboriginal thought (cf. Battiste & Henderson, 2000; James, 2001; Battiste, 2002; Nadasdy, 2003; Fixico, 2003; Waters, 2004). The Maori scholar Royal (Cunningham, 2003) suggests that there are not only two epistemologies (as suggested by Nisbett), but three basic, different systems of knowledge in the world: while Western (Judaeo-Christian) epistemology locates knowledge externally in a metaphysical system, and Eastern views situate knowledge internally, accessible via meditation and other insight practices, Indigenous epistemologies are said to offer a "third way," integrating nature and culture as one seamless system. While one may disagree whether there exist two, three, or many more different kinds of knowledge, and whether these differences are absolute or a matter of degree, it seems defensible to assume that what counts as knowledge in one place may not necessarily count as knowledge in another. In the following we will examine similarities and differences between Western and Indigenous knowledge in some more detail.

In the Western tradition, Aristotle developed rules of logic that were meant to help distinguish "true" knowledge from mistaken beliefs. This distinction between knowledge and belief is one of the cornerstones of "Judaeo-Graeco-

Roma-Christian-Renaissance-Enlightenment-Romanticist" thought (Rorty 1987, p. 57) and of the "scientific method" aiming to perfect the work of sorting epistemic wheat from chaff. Knowledge was deemed "true" if it was found to be true independent of context, that is, universally true. Such universal knowledge could then be transported from one place and dropped off at another (for example, from Ottawa to some First Nations community) without losing any of its authority. According to this account, then, the problems of declaring what is to be deemed as real knowledge, and working out how it is to be generalized and shared, are identical. If something is decided to be truly true, then it is equally true everywhere at once. There could, of course, be some local differences that may require efforts at more appropriate communication and translation—but these differences would be assumed to be minor and pragmatic, remote from the question of what is true or false.

In principle, there is nothing about this Western conception of knowledge just outlined that would prevent the possibility that there might well be Indigenous knowledge claims—claims that could be deemed to be true and shared universally. After all, much of Western research is driven by curiosity and begins locally, in scattered scientific communities. In the same way, one could very well imagine Aboriginal communities and cultures as sites of bona fide knowledge production. From the brisk sales of "Lakota Natural Formula" and other reputed "indigenous" remedies (some of which are now protected as cultural "properties") to the recent focus on an ecology that addresses the interrelations between humans and the environment ("the land"), there seem to be many possibilities.

Various impediments, however, have kept the West from taking Indigenous knowledge seriously. For one, the differences between Aboriginal and Western cultures have sometimes been reduced to a matter of orality versus literacy. Quite famously, Ong (1990; see also Fried, 2008, p. 17) has argued that thinking in oral versus literary cultures can be seen to differ in various ways: being additive rather than hierarchical; being aggregative and repetitive rather than analytical; and appropriating life worlds in mostly situated rather than abstract ways. While parts of Ong's observations regarding the situated nature of oral (Aboriginal) cultures may ring true and will be discussed later, the situatedness of knowledge does not necessarily contradict the possibility of analytical thought. In fact, some writers have argued that Aboriginal reason is very much analytical and that it is Western thought that is limited—limited by a decontextualizing scientific materialism (Schauffler, 2003, p. 7). This limited Western materialism is said to discount the vastness and authority of a creationist "terrestrial intelligence" that is "older than time, less primitive than the rational present," and is superior to human reasoning, particularly of the Western kind with its always changing hypotheses (Hogan, 2007, pp. 11, 15, 19).

Second, contemporary Western cultures tend to equate all knowledge with technical knowledge (Habermas, 1987). However, until the time of Columbus, American Aboriginal cultures were basically on par with Western cultures regarding technological knowledge and its applications (Kidwell, 1992, p. 371). Only subsequently were Aboriginal cultures left out of the benefits of the emerging technological revolution. For most in the West the resulting technological gap has been enough to rule out the very possibility that Indigenous knowledge might be worth considering.

Finally, and most troublingly, as various contemporary post-colonial scholars (for example, Holland, Lanichotte, Skinner, & Cain, 2001) have shown, the West's systematic denigration of the possibility that Indigenous and Western knowledge might be on par can be shown to function as a collective defense against confronting the immorality of having subjugated and pillaged a whole people. In line with this collective defense, colonizing and missionizing (including what Battiste calls "cognitive imperialism" [2002, p. xvi]; or what Nandy describes as the conquest of minds [1983]) are seen as altogether permissible if those perceived as "other" (Duran & Duran, 1995; Pewewardy, 2001) can be discounted as "primitive" (Deloria, 2004, p. 3), and their beliefs disregarded as "pre-scientific" or mere "childish" superstitions (Gandhi, 1998, p. 16). Such defenses could be construed in the form of the following syllogism:

- Major Premise: All bona fide knowledge forms (that is, all true beliefs) are necessarily universal truths that, with modest tinkering, can easily be tailored to fit any local circumstance;

- Minor premise: Western technology and its associated "scientific method" yields bona fide knowledge that trumps or supercedes all more "primitive" or pre-scientific beliefs;

- Therefore: Western knowledge is truer than Indigenous knowledge, and can be legitimately generalized to apply to any and all local problems, including the so-called "Indian" problem.

This line of derogatory reasoning can lead to various conclusions, including the assumptions that there is no Indigenous knowledge worth considering and that the only appropriate kind of knowledge transfer is an exclusively "top-down" strategy. Such strategies transfer knowledge gathered and sifted at the academy and/or government level down to the front-line worker, denying the very possibility that there might be other avenues of acquiring useful knowledge through the lateral exchange of best practices among relevant users of such information—for example, among more and less successful Aboriginal communities.

The type of derogatory reasoning outlined above also fails to recognize the significant cultural differences between Canada's Aboriginal peoples. In fact, rather than forming some seamless monolith, or homogenized collection of interchangeable parts, Aboriginal peoples are, in fact, culturally extraordinarily diverse (see, for example, Deloria, 1988; Battiste & Henderson, 2000; Grant, Blake, & Teucher, 2004), and neither need nor want the same things—particularly from government. Just consider the differences in languages—since language and culture are closely related—between Canada's Aboriginal peoples: in British Columbia alone, there exist eight distinct, genetically unrelated Aboriginal language families (Shaw, 2001, p. 39ff.). Saskatchewan, as another example, has three distinct Aboriginal language families: Algonquin (Cree, Saulteaux), Athapaskan (Dene), and Siouan (Dakota, Lakota). What makes this especially remarkable is that languages as diverse as, for example, English, Russian, Iranian, and Hindi are all genetic members of just one (!) language family, Indo-European, summing up the backgrounds of the majority of immigrants to Canada. Those who stress the differences between Canada's many immigrant cultures must surely stress the differences between Aboriginal cultures. Given all of the variability among Aboriginal cultures, the likelihood that what is true for one is also true for all is impossibly remote, severely limiting the efficacy of general, top-down knowledge transfers from government.

PART TWO: "BUT HOW SHAREABLE IS INDIGENOUS KNOWLEDGE?"

Whatever the institutionalized reluctances are to accept differences between Aboriginal cultures and the possibility of legitimate Indigenous knowledge (that is, to entertain the possibility that some, if not all, Aboriginal communities might possess knowledge that is key to their own well-being), the question still remains as to whether or not such knowledge—for example, cultural knowledge concerning how to create rearing conditions that make life worth living for Aboriginal youth—can be successfully transferred from one Aboriginal community to another. What is to count as a reasonable answer to this question turns very much on the contested matter of incommensurability.

Systems of knowledge are said to be incommensurable when they pass like ships in the night, with the knowledge claims of one system having no truth values in the accounting structures of the other. Falling back into the arms of a hapless relativism, some see such incommensurabilities around every corner. Others, less willing to sell the epistemic farm, argue that while any two cultures with sufficiently different histories or life patterns will

necessarily evolve suitably different epistemologies, or frameworks of understanding, these differences need not automatically work at conceptual cross-
purposes, and could, under proper circumstances, be made to approach one
another at some metaphysical or other tangent. For example, Western and
Chinese philosophies have been changing over time and were never homogeneous: the Greek philosopher Heraclitus can be said to have been rather
"Eastern," while his counterpart, the Chinese philosopher Mo-Tzu, was quite
"Western" (Nisbett 2003, p. 29f.). Heidegger's later philosophical writings
certainly celebrate contextual thinking involving "the land," as well as a turn
from instrumental technology and knowledge production to a rather cre-
ative "techne" and "episteme" in a revelatory sense (Heidegger, 1993). Today,
in a time of globalization that affects research and research practices, different epistemologies can be seen to adopt modifications from each other (Nisbett, 2003, p. 41).

Similarly, it might very well prove to be true that Indigenous epistemologies are importantly different from both Western and Eastern conceptions
of knowing. Such differences could help to explain the poor record enjoyed
by traditional "top-down" strategies of knowledge transfer. And yet, none of
these differences would necessarily seem to pose a threat to the serious possibility of sharing knowledge between various Indigenous communities
themselves. However, what would present such a problem, particularly to
epidemiological research, would be any claim that Indigenous knowledge
itself is so varied that its wide-ranging forms are themselves incommensurable.
While no one seems particularly committed to imagining that each and every
band or individual Aboriginal is necessarily locked into an inescapable "other
minds" problem, there is an important and recurring claim in the contemporary literature that could, in the worst case, easily amount to the same thing.
The issue at stake here concerns the degree to which Aboriginal knowing is
understood to be wholly situated, or place-specific, as a consequence of its
natural ties to the land. Indeed, various contemporary Aboriginal scholars
have strongly emphasized a relationship between place and knowledge as an
example of the difference that divides Western and Native epistemic practices.
For example, Battiste and Henderson (2000) have characterized this difference between Western and Native scientific practices, with regard to ecological knowledge, as follows:

> [t]he traditional ecological knowledge of Indigenous peoples is sci-
> entific, in the sense that it is empirical, experimental, and systematic.
> It differs in two important aspects from Western science, however:
> traditional ecological knowledge is highly localized and it is social.

Its focus is the web of relationships between humans, animals, plants, natural forces, spirits, and land forms in a particular locality, as opposed to the discovery of universal 'laws.' (p. 44ff.)

On this account, Western and Indigenous epistemologies are seen to differ principally with regard to the presumed existence of an inherent relationship between cultural practices and the specifics of the natural environment (Canada-Royal Commission on Aboriginal Peoples, 1996, Vol. 4, p. 454). As the anthropologist Crisca Bierwert (1999) notes, for example, Northwest Coast Salish people's myths trace the emanation of their ancestors to local lands that are understood as inherently imbued with agentic sacred beings and features (p. 40). As such, Indigenous concepts of place are often said to be permeated with essences and meanings that are not perceived as culturally constructed, but as actually preceding human culture (Bierwert, 1999, p. 39). Within such accounting systems, "place" has both a social and a moral impact; it is not only a repository, but also a source of knowledge (Bierwert, 1999, pp. 41, 43). It follows from such views that changes in the local ecosystem imply changes in a community's identity and social relations. The loss of a watershed, for example, can be seen to cause a loss of embodied memories and identity (Battiste & Henderson, 2000, p. 42). Taken together, these observations draw attention to a hypothesized place-specific constraint upon Indigenous knowledge in its localized forms, a view according to which knowledge can be seen as inherently "belonging" to particular places.

Given such place-specific forms of knowledge, while a band may treat knowledge offered by a neighbouring band with respect, it may view such knowledge as not applicable to its own situated contexts, and therefore as not shareable. This place-specific constraint appears to apply particularly to bands on North America's west coast that gain their livelihood mainly through fishing. These communities may be able to trace their "absolute and eternal beginning" back to particular places, in fact, more or less the same area where they are living now, celebrating these origins in their communal narrative histories (Brody, 2004, p. 15). In contrast, as Brody points out, Native hunting peoples, even within British Columbia's northwest areas, have traditionally been more mobile, using many different resources and living sites, and do not necessarily believe that they originated in the areas in which they are living today. Thus, traditional hunting peoples may have less attachment to specific areas of land, although this does not mean that they feel less strongly than other peoples about the land and its resources (p. 15f.). The relations with "the land" are, of course, much more troubled among most North American Native peoples east of the Rocky Mountains: as the colonizers set foot in the east and moved westwards, they drove out entire Native peoples who, themselves fleeing westwards, dislocated in a chain reaction other Native peoples even before these had made contact with the colonizers. For example, the westward-moving Cree dislocated the Beaver people further west towards the Peace River headwaters in Alberta, with the Beaver themselves dispersing the Sekani into the Rocky Mountains (Brody, 2004, p. 23). Similarly, the Lenape (Delaware) who, according to legend, had sold Manhattan to the Dutch, were driven into Ohio and Indiana and, from there, on to Arkansas, Kansas, Texas, and Oklahoma (Schutt, 2007). The flight of chief Sitting Bull and his Lakota tribe into Canada is well-documented, and Dakota and Lakota people still live in southern Saskatchewan and Saskatoon today (Palmer, 2008). Nevertheless, all of these peoples' associations with "the land" remain central, albeit in apparently less absolute ways than among Northwest Coast fishing peoples.

A "search for the importance of place" is also not uncommon in Western culture. However, in Western thought, "place" has usually been associated with subjection (cf. God's advice to Adam and Eve to subdue the earth [Genesis 1: 28]) and territorial ownership (Simpson, 2000), no matter whether in capitalist or communist systems (Marcuse, 1989). Perhaps as a consequence of the West's troubled history of territorial wars and repeated expulsions, contemporary Western culture and its scholars also often categorize memories, identities, and even epistemological conceptions of place in terms of their situatedness in local "spaces," but view these notions of "space" as intellectually or culturally constituted. Unlike their Indigenous colleagues, Western scholars commonly have strong reservations about imbuing space—or place—with any essentialist, never mind pre-cultural, significance. Particularly post-colonial scholars, who are among the most committed to the contextualized nature of knowledge, often equate such essentialist ideas with the contested notions of "homelands" and "ethnic purity," and emphasize instead a terminology (for example, "site," "situated," "positioned") that draws attention to what is perceived as the cultural construction of place (McDowell & Sharp, 1997). For example, Gupta and Ferguson stress that "all associations of place, people, and culture are social and historical creations to be explained, not given natural facts" (1977, p. 4). In apparent contrast, then, to at least some Indigenous beliefs, most Western views exclude the possibility that humans and their knowledge literally "belong" to any one place. In a simplified sense, the differences could perhaps be summed up in this way: according to Western views, humans take for granted that they can own and instrumentalize the earth for their needs and for human knowledge construction; while Aboriginal views stress that it is the earth that owns and brings forth knowledge and humans. However, it would seem to be a mistake to identify Aboriginal sensitivities to, and cultural knowledge of, place and spiritual essences as "static," since constant flux is one of the central features in many Aboriginal philosophies (e.g., Battiste and Henderson, 2000; Little Bear, 2002; Waters, 2004).

At best, all of this leaves open a critical list of questions for epidemiologists, particularly in British Columbia: if, as scholars of Aboriginal thought have stressed, traditional Indigenous knowledge is place-specific, and if, as a consequence, policies cannot be safely generalized beyond a particular community's boundaries, can there be any basis for sharing cultural knowledge? In short, with its emphasis on local place, can Indigenous knowledge be generalized? At least for some, the answer appears to be an unqualified "no." According to Little Bear (2000), for example, even an individual within a community can never know for certain what someone else knows, given the flux and complexity of the local ecosystem (p. 80).

Nevertheless, there are evident exceptions to such wholly situated notions of knowledge-sharing. For example, there would seem to be certain knowledge claims that are indeed shared and taught across a large variety of North American Aboriginal communities with presumably differing epistemologies, including, for example, the claims that nature and culture are inherently interrelated, that knowledge is based on concrete experience, verified by personal memories, and even (perhaps paradoxically) the very claim, widely shared, that knowledge and its narratives are place-specific (Little Bear, 2002, p. 80; see also Battiste & Henderson, 2000, pp. 42–44). More importantly, for almost two decades, Aboriginal Elders from all over Canada, including the communities on the West Coast that are most place-sensitive, have been meeting annually to exchange knowledge and, more recently, to hold workshops with the aim of helping their communities heal. While these Elders come from widely diverging places, their meetings are self-understood as necessitated by what amounts to a common plight imposed by colonization and its damaging effects. Such common post-contact circumstances, it would seem, are widely understood to warrant a common response and to open the possibility for lateral knowledge transfers between different Aboriginal communities.

In this and the previous section, we have worked out some of the similarities and differences between Indigenous and Western knowledge systems, as well as the place-specificity of Indigenous knowledges. In our final part we now want to summarize our research on Aboriginal youth suicide in British Columbia. This research exemplifies the need for epidemiological work at the band level.

PART THREE: THE MYTH OF YOUTH SUICIDE
AS AN ENDEMIC ABORIGINAL PROBLEM

In light of all of the apparent differences between Aboriginal cultures within Canada, our own research group has grown deeply skeptical of generic accounts of the Aboriginal condition, particularly when these serve to promote overgeneralized, one-size-fits-all accounts of national suicide rates. In the process of pursuing these concerns, we have focused on three points. First, instead of uncritically accepting the received view that high rates of suicide are somehow characteristic of the whole of Aboriginal life in Canada, we have so far systematically examined (one community at a time) the rates of youth suicide in each of British Columbia's almost 200 First Nations bands. Looking back over a 13-year period of data collection, we have found that almost 90 percent of British Columbia's bands are remarkably free of youth suicides, while the lion's share of all reported suicides occurred in only 10 percent of the bands (Chandler, Lalonde, Sokol, & Hallett, 2003). These numbers clearly demonstrate that youth suicide is not a problem for many British Columbia bands, although it is indeed a devastating problem for a small minority of communities.

Second, we have worked to better understand the particular ways in which Aboriginal youth meet with the dramatic changes typical of adolescence and have found that their ways of doing so differ importantly from those of their age-mates from non-Aboriginal cultures. Adolescence is a developmental period when young people first become aware of the flow of time in their lives: while younger children live in a near-timeless world, adolescents are beginning to understand the challenge to somehow create some kind of personal continuity of self despite one's obvious changes in time. Earlier research by Chandler and Ball (1990) had suggested that adolescents are more likely to commit suicide when they find themselves unable to successfully link up their past, present, and future into some coherent account of self-continuity. Building on this work, we approached two Aboriginal bands in British Columbia (one urban, one rural and remote), as well as a comparison group of mostly Euro-Canadian adolescents. We presented our young participants with various abbreviated comic book versions of narratives common in West Coast Aboriginal or Euro-Canadian cultures. For example, some of the comics featured main characters such as Bear Woman (from a traditional West Coast Aboriginal story), or Jean Valjean (from Victor Hugo's Les Misérables). These characters all share in the experience of having changed remarkably through some dramatic event—while still somehow remaining the same. Our questions to our participants asked how it was possible for these characters to have changed and yet be the same; based on these discussions we then asked our participants about change and sameness in their own lives.

The findings have been discussed in extensive detail elsewhere (Chandler, Lalonde, Sokol, & Hallett, 2003; Chandler, Lalonde, & Teucher, 2003). In short, most non-Aboriginal youth argued for some core of individual essence (for example, fingerprints, personality, soul) that would not change over time and thereby connects past, present, and future. In contrast, most of our Aboriginal participants—from both our participating communities—did not rely on some sense of timeless personal essence but, instead, told stories that traced a flux of personal changes at different times of their lives, always in the context of networks of relations (parents, kinship, friends). With our young Aboriginal participants it seemed to be the very act of telling these changes that knitted together time slices in past, present, and future into a narrative. In other words, most non-Aboriginal adolescents built their accounts on the presumed existence of a timeless self, while most Aboriginal adolescents laid out a self that changes through time and context. Based on these findings we then hypothesized, with regard to our Aboriginal adolescents, that there had to be an important connection between the individual ways that these young people arrived at a sense of personal continuity and how well their bands had been able to maintain or re-establish a shared sense of cultural continuity. In other words, if some bands had lost relevant amounts of cultural knowledge and social continuity, due to the effects of colonialism, then it might be harder for such bands to convey a sense of personal continuity to their young people— a continuity that relies on a strong link between personal and social matters.

Third, we set out to specify what it is that especially characterizes those bands with markedly higher and lower youth suicide rates. Building on our hypothesis that those bands that have maintained or re-established a sense of cultural continuity somehow make it possible for their youth to find their lives worth living, the question arose: what kind of cultural markers could help fashion a sense of cultural continuity? We proposed eight such markers of cultural continuity and tabulated their presence or absence for every band in British Columbia. These markers included: a) evidence that particular bands had taken steps to secure Aboriginal title to their traditional lands; b) evidence of having reclaimed certain rights of self-government from provincial and federal governments; c) presence of educational services (for example, schools); d) availability of police and fire protection services; e) presence of health delivery services; f) existence of cultural facilities (for example, Long/Big Houses, community centres) to help preserve and enact cultural practices; g) participation of women in local governance (a historical feature in British Columbia); and h) the existence of child and family services within a community. As it turned out, suicide rates are lowest or even zero in those communities that have most or all of these markers in place, and highest in those that have few or even none of these markers present. Among all the markers, however, the achievement of self-government is clearly the strongest single factor and predictor of suicide rates in British Columbia (for more details see Chandler, Lalonde, Sokol, & Hallett, 2003). The exact causal relationship between the presence or absence of these cultural continuity factors and the incidence of youth suicide is not yet known, but further studies are underway, attempting to establish the extent of actual youth involvement in Aboriginal communities.

What is already absolutely clear from these epidemiological studies is that youth suicide is not a typical feature of Aboriginal cultures and that many Aboriginal communities are indeed well equipped to rear their youth in ways such that they find life worth living (Lalonde & Chandler, 2008). These Aboriginal bands possess various kinds of Indigenous knowledge that provide their young people with a connection to their past, present, and as yet unrealized future. If this knowledge could be articulated, made explicit, and shared between bands, perhaps the bands with high suicide rates might stand to benefit.

With regard to our ongoing research, we have been devising further studies meant to examine the extent of actual youth involvement in Aboriginal cultural activities at the band level. One study already underway compares cultural similarities and differences in self-knowledge between children from Nottingham (UK), Osaka (Japan), and different Cree communities in Saskatchewan. Another research project in Saskatchewan proposes to study the relationship between Aboriginal youths' "civic identity" (participation in communal practices) in different communities as a marker of their social and personal health. We hope that, together, the findings will shed more light on cultural forms of knowledge, as well as the possibilities, the potential limits, and the impact of knowledge transfers on local communities in various Indigenous cultures in an interconnected world (Smith & Ward, 2000). Yet it is precisely this possibility of "lateral" knowledge-sharing of "best practices" between communities that governments (with their preference for top-down knowledge transfers) regularly ignore. With regard to Aboriginal youth suicide, top-down knowledge transfers go hand in hand with traditional epidemiological research that has supplied government with suicide rates calculated indiscriminately across the whole of Canada. By contrast, future epidemiological research that is respectful of differences—between Western and Indigenous epistemologies as well as between Aboriginal cultures—and of potential, place-specific incommensurabilities of knowledge between individual bands can advance lateral knowledge-sharing practices that address existing health disparities more adequately at individual band levels and may provide more effective solutions for those communities that are struggling with high suicide rates.

Our findings regarding Aboriginal systems of knowledge and their differences from Western knowledge systems, as well as the cultural differences between Canada's Aboriginal peoples, are useful not only for our studies of Aboriginal youth suicide rates in British Columbia; they are also helping us to better understand a variety of social health concerns among Aboriginal children and adolescents elsewhere in Canada, including Aboriginal children's conceptions of self-knowledge, as well as the shaping of Aboriginal youths' civic identities to the extent that they participate, and are included, in the activities of their communities. Moreover, our findings promise to be useful for epidemiological studies that aim to understand Aboriginal health in a wider sense, including the incidence of birth defects, infant death, and diabetes, and the variations of such health concerns between individual bands. By gathering knowledge at the band level, by building on the cultural knowledge that exists, in varying degrees, within Aboriginal communities, and by championing lateral knowledge transfers between communities, we are, in effect, suggesting a new overall approach to Aboriginal population health research.

In this chapter we have grappled with a number of dilemmas facing epidemiologists, surrounding the contested status of "Indigenous knowledge." First, we have tried to bring out a tension between distinctive cultural constructions of knowledge. One of these, rooted in Western European intellectual traditions, understands "true" belief to be a form of technical knowledge that is context independent and inherently generalizable. By these lights the only conceivable form of legitimate knowledge transfer involves a "top-down" process by means of which Western "scientific" knowledge is filtered down to Indigenous groups—groups that are seen to be poorly positioned to ever make serious contributions to the generation and transfer of real knowledge. In contrast, certain scholars of aboriginality have promoted a second and more situated view that includes the possibility of naturally contextualized or place-specific knowledge forms. On this second account, claims in favour of universalizable knowledge are often viewed with suspicion, and reacted to as a further attempt to colonize the minds of Aboriginal people. Although potentially conducive to promoting a more lateral or community-to-community form of knowledge transfer between Aboriginal groups, the good prospects of such exchanges of "best practices"—especially with regard to Aboriginal health (and not limited to youth suicide)—would appear to depend upon identifying some "stop rule," a rule that successfully preserves the place of "place" without so locking each and every Native community into a kind of context-specific solitude that excludes the very possibility of any meaningful form of knowledge transfer. We suggest that the shared "plight" suffered by Canada's First Nations and other Aboriginal groups offers sufficient common ground to allow for the real possibility of sharing such Indigenous knowledge forms.

Authors' note: I am most grateful to Dr. Michael Chandler at the University of British Columbia for his many suggestions in the development of this chapter. I also wish to acknowledge the fellowship support from the Canadian Institutes of Health Research (CIHR) and the Michael Smith Foundation (MSFHR).

REFERENCES

Battiste, M., & Youngblood Henderson, J. (2000). *Protecting Indigenous knowledge and heritage: A global challenge.* Saskatoon: Purich Publishing.

Battiste, M. (Ed.). (2002). *Reclaiming Indigenous voice and vision.* Vancouver: UBC Press.

Bierwert, C. (1999). *Brushed by cedar, living by the river: Coast Salish figures of power.* Tucson: University of Arizona Press.

Brody, H. (2004). *Maps and dreams: Indians and the British Columbia frontier.* Vancouver, BC: Douglas & McIntyre.

Canada. Royal Commission on Aboriginal Peoples (1996). *Report of the Royal Commission on Aboriginal Peoples, Vol. 4.* Ottawa, ON: The Commission.

Chandler, M. J., & Ball, L. (1990). Continuity and commitment: A developmental analysis of the identity formation process in suicidal and non-suicidal youth. In H. Bosma & S. Jackson (Eds.), *Coping and self-concept in adolescence* (pp. 149–166). New York: Springer-Verlag.

Chandler, M. J., Lalonde, C. E., Sokol, B., & Hallett, D. (2003). *Personal persistence, identity development, and suicide.* Monographs of the Society for Research in Child Development. Boston: Blackwell.

Chandler, M. J., Lalonde, C. E., & Teucher, U. (2003). Culture, continuity, and the limits of narrativity: A comparison of the self-narratives of Native and Non-Native youth. In C. Lightfoot & C. Daiuth (Eds.), *Narrative analysis: Studying the development of individuals in society* (pp. 245–265). Thousand Oaks, CA: Sage.

Chandler, M. J., and Lalonde, C. E. (2008). Cultural Continuity as a moderator of suicide risk among Canada's First Nations. In L. Kirmayer & G. Valaskakis (Eds.), *Healing traditions: The mental health of Aboriginal peoples in Canada.* Vancouver: UBC Press.

Cunningham, C. (2003). Indigenous by definition, experience, or world view. *BMJ, 327*, 403–404.

Deloria, V. (1988). *Custer died for your sins—an Indian manifesto.* Norman, OK: University of Oklahoma Press.

Deloria, V. (2004). Philosophy and the tribal peoples. In A. Waters (Ed.). *American Indian thought: Philosophical essays* (pp. 3–11). Malden, MA: Blackwell Publishing.

Duran, E., & Duran, B. (1995). *Native American postcolonial psychology.* Albany: State University of New York Press.

Fixico, D. F. (2003). *The American Indian mind in a linear world: American Indian studies and traditional knowledge.* New York: Routledge.

Fried, J. (2008). *Das Mittelalter: Geschichte und Kultur.* Munich: C. H. Beck.

Gandhi, L. (1998). *Postcolonial theory: A critical introduction.* New York: Columbia University Press.

Grant, L., Blake, J. S., & Teucher, U. C. (2004). Meanings of Musqueam ancestral names: The Capilano tradition. *University of British Columbia working papers in linguistics:* UBCWPL, *14,* 45–66.

Gupta, A., & Ferguson, J. (Eds). (1997). *Culture power place: Explorations in critical anthropology.* Durham: Duke University.

Habermas, J. (1987). *The philosophical discourse of modernity.* (F. Lawrence, Trans.). Cambridge, MA: MIT Press. (Original work published 1985).

Health Canada (2006). *First Nations, Inuit, and Aboriginal health.* Accessed February 16, 2009. http://www.hc-sc.gc.ca/fniah-spnia/promotion/suicide/index-eng.php

Heidegger, M. (1993). Building, dwelling, thinking; The question concerning technology. In D. F. Krell (Ed.), *Martin Heidegger: Basic writings.* New York: HarperCollins.

Hofstede, G. (1980). *Culture's consequences: International differences in work-related values.* Beverly Hills: Sage.

Hogan, L. (2007). *Dwellings: A spiritual history of the living world.* New York: W. W. Norton & Company.

Holland, D., Lanichotte, W., Skinner, D., & Cain, C. (2001). *Identity and agency in cultural worlds.* Cambridge, MA: Harvard University Press.

James, K. (Ed). (2001). *Science and Native American communities.* Lincoln: University of Nebraska Press.

Kidwell, C. S. (1992). Systems of knowledge. In A. M. Josephy, Jr. (Ed.), *America in 1492: The world of the Indian peoples before the arrival of Columbus* (pp. 369–403). New York: Alfred A. Knopf.

Kirmayer, L. (1994). Suicide among Canadian aboriginal people. *Transcultural Psychiatric Research Review, 31,* 3–57.

Little Bear, L. (2002). Jagged worldviews colliding. In M. Battiste (Ed.), *Reclaiming Indigenous voice and vision* (pp. 39–49). Vancouver: UBC Press.

Marcuse. H. (1989). *Counterrevolution and revolt.* Boston, MA: Beacon Press.

Markus, H. R., & Kitayama, S. (1991). Culture and the self: Implications for cognition, emotion, and motivation. *Psychological Review, 98,* 224–253.

McDowell, L., & Sharp, J. (Eds). (1997). *Space, gender, knowledge: Feminist readings.* London: Arnold.

Nadasdy, P. (2003). *Hunters and bureaucrats: Power, knowledge, and aboriginal-state relations in the southwest Yukon.* Vancouver: UBC Press.

Nandy, A. (1983). *The intimate enemy: Loss and recovery of self under colonialism.* Delhi: Oxford University Press.

Nisbett, R. E. (2003). *The geography of thought: How Asians and Westerners think differently... and why.* New York: Free Press.

Nisbett, R. E., Peng, K., Choi, I., & Norenzayan, A. (2001). Culture and systems of thought: Holistic versus analytic cognition. *Psychological Review, 108*(2), 291–310.

Ong, W. (1990). *Orality and literacy: The technologizing of the world.* New York: Routledge.

Palmer, J. D. (2008). *Dakota people: A history of the Dakota, Lakota and Nakota through 1863.* Jefferson, NC: McFarland & Company.

Pewewardy, C. (2001). Indigenous consciousness, education, and science: Issues of perception and language. In K. James (Ed.). *Science and Native American communities: Legacies of pain, visions of promise* (pp. 16–21). Lincoln: University of Nebraska Press.

Rorty, A. O. (1987). Persons as rhetorical categories. *Social Research, 54*(1), 55–72.

Sallot, J. (2004, September 14). Aboriginals to receive $700-million. *The Globe and Mail,* p. A5.

Schauffler, E. M. (2003). *Turning to earth: Stories of ecological conversion.* Charlottesville: University of Virginia Press.

Schutt, A. C. (2007). *Peoples of the river valleys: The odyssey of the Delaware Indians.* Philadelphia: University of Pennsylvania Press.

Shaw, P. (2001). Language and identity, language and the land. B.C. *Studies, 131,* 39–55.

Simpson, J. W. (2002). *Yearning for the land: A search for the importance of place.* New York: Pantheon Books.

Smith, C., & Ward, G. K. (2000). *Indigenous cultures in an interconnected world.* Vancouver: UBC Press.

Triandis, H. C. (1995). *Individualism and collectivism.* Boulder, Westview Press.

Waters, A. (Ed.). (2004). *American Indian thought: Philosophical essays.* Malden, MA: Blackwell Publishing.

The Shifting Discourse of "Public Participation": Implications in Changing Models of Health System Regionalization

Kelly Chessie

A midst an ethos of fiscal restraint and retrenchment, the 1980s and 1990s saw Western nations questioning the goals of their welfare states, including health systems and publicly funded health care (Crichton et al., 1997; Drache & Sullivan, 1999). As health care costs and service demands climbed alongside falling tax revenues, and as questions grew regarding sustainability and imbalanced resource allocations amongst public sectors, governments introduced reforms to restructure and rationalize health care delivery (Wetzel, 2005).

Echoing the moves of the international scene, and situated within broader neo-liberal transformations of the welfare state, Canada and its provinces turned their attention to health systems, and governments announced commissions to comb their systems for efficiencies. Many themes emerged within the commissions' reports, including encouragement to adopt a broader definition of health, to increase attention to illness prevention and health promotion, and to shift from institutional-based care to community-based care where feasible (Mhatre & Deber, 1992). Another theme was a call for greater public involvement and community engagement in health system planning and governance (Mhatre & Deber, 1992; Crichton et al., 1997). Citing population health and community development logics (such as the Ottawa Charter), calling on legitimation needs and increased public accountability, and referencing responsible citizenship, the reports recommended increased public participation as one part of multi-faceted health reform strategies (e.g., Hyndman, 1989; Murray, 1990; Nova Scotia Commission on Health Care, 1989; Rochon, 1987; Seaton, 1991).

On the heels of the reviews, nine provinces and the Northwest Territories introduced, or reintroduced,[1] policies to regionalize their systems. These policies, while differing from province to province in their specifics, shared two generalities. First, they devolved varying levels of power from provincial ministries down to newly created sub-provincial authorities, each of which would be overseen by a governance board comprised of local community members (Kouri, Chessie, & Lewis, 2002). Second, the policies eliminated the many independent health facility boards that had until then been operating throughout the communities, thus, in effect, centralizing their powers up to the newly created regional boards (Lewis, 1997; Lomas, 1999; Rasmussen, 2001).

The publicly stated intentions for regionalization included not only structural, but also substantive, changes to governance models through greater involvement of citizens and communities. This shift to include public voices in health system governance (alongside those of traditional players such as health care providers, administrators, policy-makers, and governments) led regionalization to be cited as the most radical reform to Canadian health care since the introduction of medicare (Lomas, 1996; Lomas, Woods, & Veenstra, 1997).

Within a decade of these announcements, a subsequent wave of reform swept across Canada, and while most governments remained committed to regionalization, they announced adjustments to the models. These included reductions in the number of regions, altered board compositions (for example, some provinces eliminated elections in favour of appointments), and clarifications to accountabilities and authorities between regions and governments (e.g., Clair, 2001; Fyke, 2001; Mazankowski, 2001; Saskatchewan Health, 2001).

Another wave of reform is now cresting, and with it we have seen Prince Edward Island disband its authorities (Prince Edward Island Ministry of Health, 2006), New Brunswick merge its eight regions into two (New Brunswick, 2008), and Alberta re-centralize its nine boards to one (Liepert, 2008). There is speculation that Saskatchewan's authorities are also being reconsidered. Manitoba, on the other hand, has received a favourable review of its regions with recommendations that the province devolve more authority (Gray, Delaquis, & Closson, 2008), and Ontario announced "integrated networks" (LHINs) (Government of Ontario, 2006), a possible tentative step towards regionalization.

Despite these shifts and repositionings, and despite the early stated significance of these boards (e.g., Lomas, 1996; Lomas, Woods, & Veenstra, 1997), we have seen relatively little critical attention paid to the changing policies. The Canadian literature has produced largely atheoretical, descriptive reviews and polls (e.g., Frankish et al., 1999; Kouri, Chessie, & Lewis, 2002; Lomas, Woods, & Veenstra, 1997; Lomas, Veenstra, & Woods, 1997a;

1997b; Marchildon, 2005). This is especially the case when considering the amended governance models of the second and third waves of regionalization, and when considering the substantive goals of public participation and community engagement in health system governance.

Using Saskatchewan as a case study, this paper presents an analysis of key government texts that introduced the 1992 policies and their 2001 amendments. In particular, it attends to their discourses of "public participation" and "community engagement," noting the ways "publics" were positioned into the models, the expectations contained within these positions, the roles and assumptions that support the shifts, and the tensions and contradictions that appear across the texts.

Although situated in Saskatchewan, this case study has relevance beyond its borders. Regionalization exists in various forms nationally and internationally (e.g., Deber, 1996; Dwyer, 2004; Kouri, Chessie, & Lewis, 2002; Marchildon, 2005; Wetzel, 2005). Furthermore, as Abelson et al. (2003) write, public participation ideologies have gripped the health care system. As Saskatchewan is poised to enter another round of health reform, and as shifts in governance models continue across the nation, stepping back to analyze the public policy discourses within which these shifts are embedded—and the implications contained therein—is timely work. These analyses add insight as to the changing nature of our public roles and the changing ways we are to relate to political and administrative systems.

In the case of the Saskatchewan texts, the 1992 discourses—heavy in logics of public participation and community engagement as routes to empowerment and accountability, and calling on the political rights and capacities of citizens and communities to participate in local health system governance—give way to new logics in the 2001 texts. In the 2001 text, we see discourses that call on logics of expertise and technocratic concerns and that insert "publics," but in restricted capacities, as individuals and patients with input and advice to offer to planning experts and decision makers. These shifts in the discourses are significant and carry with them implications for publics, communities, policy-makers, administrators, and practitioners that merit our consideration. As Hansen (2003) reminded us in his comparison of Saskatchewan tax policies: "Words and expressions do not just represent our world but also help to construct it. Language and action are closely intertwined" (p. 9).

THEORETICAL FRAMEWORKS AND METHODS
Public participation and community engagement in health system governance have been argued along many lines, including state-democratization, legitimation and public accountability, and community development and empower-

ment logics (e.g., Church et al., 2002; Dickinson, 2004; Hyndman, 1989; Lomas, 1999; MacKinnon, 2006; Murray, 1990; Rochon, 1987; Seaton, 1991; Side & Keefe, 2004; Veenstra & Lomas, 1999; World Health Organization, 1986). Public participation theorists and evaluators have cautioned us to clarify the goals and intentions of participation (Abelson et al., 2003; Baggott, 2005; Church et al., 2002; Davies, Wetherell, & Barnett, 2006; Morgan, 2001; Scutchfield, Ireson, & Hall, 2004; Taylor, Wilkinson, & Cheers, 2006). Models of public participation have been articulated that situate participants to attend to micro-, meso-, and macro-level discussions on services, systems, and governance policies, and along continuums ranging from passive receipt of information, to simple provision of input, to shared power and decision-making, as experts, consumers, patients, clients, taxpayers, or citizens (e.g., Arnstein, 1969; Charles & DeMaio, 1993; Collins & Evans, 2002; Tritter & McCallum, 2006).

Informed by these broad theoretical frameworks and their notions of differing roles, differing levels of engagements, and differing contributions, key documents detailing the 1992 introduction of and 2001 amendments to governance models in Saskatchewan were analyzed using methods of critical discourse analysis (Fairclough, 1989; Rogers, 2004; Wodak & Meyer, 2001). In keeping with this methodology, the current analysis moves beyond the description and specific details of the texts to consider the frameworks and ideas that lie behind the specified details.

Two guiding questions anchored the readings of the documents. First, *where* do we see "publics" and "communities" called upon and inserted into decision-making and governance models? Second, within this subset of text, *how* are "publics" and "communities" called upon? That is, *in what capacity, with what means,* and *to what ends* are they inserted into the health care governance and decision-making processes? Where can we read more democratically rooted intentions, positioning participants as decision-making publics, citizens, and representatives of collective social and community interests? Where do we see population health logics being called on, wherein people have the opportunity to control decisions affecting their health and the health of their communities? Where do we hear more technocratic-informed intentions that insert public participants as individuals, patients, consumers, and clients, only providing input to those who make the decisions in the planning and delivery of satisfying care?

For both the 1992 and 2001 models, the government publications that detailed their announcements and the publicly stated intentions for the reforms and their new governance models were analyzed. There were three such documents for the 1992 model (Saskatchewan Health, 1992a; 1992b; 1992c) and one for the 2001 model (Saskatchewan Health, 2001).

As Smith (1990) reminds us, these texts "entered the public textual discourse at a particular moment in local political history" (p. 25). To contextualize these government publications, a broader series of texts were thus considered. These included the commission reports released prior to each of the reforms (the 1990 Murray Commission[2] and the 2001 Fyke Commission); the Hansard transcripts for the month preceding and following the August 17, 1992, announcement (Legislative Assembly of Saskatchewan, 1992a)[3]; and the Throne Speeches that opened and prorogued the relevant sessions of the Saskatchewan Legislative Assemblies (Legislative Assembly of Saskatchewan, 1992b; 1993; 2001; 2002).

Secondary sources were also reviewed to help more fully to understand the local political environment within which these announcements were being made (e.g., Adams, 2001; McIntosh & Marchildon, forthcoming; Rasmussen, 2001; Wetzel, 2005). From these texts, we are reminded that Saskatchewan's health reforms were anchored within parallel national and international movements and were heavily influenced by an ethos of fiscal constraint, debt reduction, and welfare state and service reconfigurations and retractions. As well, health reforms were happening within a field ripe with commission reports and system reviews that advised change and restructuring. In tandem with the restraints and contractions, the Saskatchewan reforms of the 1990s were argued within goals of advancement and extension of the T. C. Douglas medicare model, such that the publicly funded system would not only remove financial barriers to access, but would also be restructured so as to orient to "wellness."

Both the 1992 and the 2001 policies were announced by a New Democratic Party government. In October of 1991, the NDP had returned to power as a majority government, ending a 10-year reign of the Conservative Party who would now serve as their opposition. The 2001 announcements, however, were made midway through the NDP's third term, when it had returned as a minority government and had formed a governing alliance with the Liberal Party.

The broader package of the Saskatchewan health reforms of the 1990s (for example, hospital closures in rural Saskatchewan, budget reductions, and de-insuring of dental care), of which regionalization was but one element, were fodder for much political debate and critique. Added to this, not long into the 1992 governance model, the government prevented and reversed several contentious health district decisions, damaging relations with the boards (McIntosh & Marchildon, forthcoming). Despite the stated intentions of the 1992 policies to devolve power to communities and their boards, this interference seemed to counter their stated logics.

According to McIntosh and Marchildon (forthcoming), the health reform backlash, coupled with the need for further reforms and a stated concern for the viability of medicare in Canada, led then NDP Premier Roy Romanow to announce a new Saskatchewan health care commission in 2000. The Fyke Commission was to review the system, identifying challenges and areas for improvement, and recommending strategies for sustainability. Fyke reported in April 2001, to then NDP Premier Lorne Calvert.⁴ The commission's recommendations were many, but of particular relevance here are its recommendations to amalgamate health districts (to increase their overall size and thus their available infrastructure and personnel resources), clarify the responsibilities and relationships of the boards and the ministry, and, if voter turnout remained low, consider alternatives to public elections as a means of selecting board members.

Shortly after Fyke reported, the Minister of Health (having completed an additional round of consultations through the Standing Committee on Health Care) announced amendments to the 1992 policy. Among them was the amalgamation of the 32 health districts into 12 regions, and replacing their district health boards with Regional Health Authorities (RHAS). Elections were eliminated, and boards would now be fully appointed through the ministry and Lieutenant-Governor. Community Advisory Networks (CANS) were introduced as formal—albeit optional and with unspecified terms of reference—structures to link communities with Regional Health Authorities and to support community involvement in the setting of priorities (Saskatchewan Health, 2001).

That being the broader political and historical context within which these four reports were announced, let us now examine the reports themselves in more detail.

THE 1992 ANNOUNCEMENTS

Three publications authored by the Ministry of Health were issued in 1992 to detail the health reforms that were underway. The first was "A Saskatchewan Vision for Health" (1992a), a four-page, 9" × 4" pamphlet written for the Saskatchewan public. The second was "A Saskatchewan Vision for Health: A Framework for Change" (1992b), a 25-page, letter-size document, written for the Saskatchewan public. It was released to the public on August 17, 1992. The third was "A Saskatchewan Vision for Health: Challenges and Opportunities" (1992c), a six-page, letter-size document, written for the Saskatchewan public. The exact dates of release for the first and third documents are not certain, although the third appears to have been issued some time after the August 1992 release of the "Framework for Change." How the three documents were distributed or how widely they may have been disseminated is not certain. Then Minister of Health Louise Simard issued all three documents.

In the upper right corner of all pages of all three documents appears a running head "Working Together Toward Wellness." As a set, the three documents are replete with references to public participation in attempts to "empower communities to work together to form health districts—to provide better health services than a single community could offer on its own" (1992a, p. 2). We read that "community-based means local control of the health system" (1992a, p. 3). The 1992 reports call on the World Health Organization definition of health (1992b, p. 2) and T. C. Douglas's two-phased approach to health care (1992b, p. 3). They state: "Today, that same community spirit of innovation and caring is needed to take the next step." They add: "This approach means the sharing of responsibility, knowledge and decision-making between communities and governments, between health care consumers and health care providers" (1992b, p. 3). We read that "communities have asked for more say in the planning and delivery of local health services" and "many health boards and health professionals are seeking ways to join forces, to share knowledge and experience" (1992c, p. 3).

Community involvement and public participation—the themes of interest in this analysis—appear in several of the strategies. The first strategy is to implement public policies that promote health, and "it is critical that public...and communities are involved" (1992b, p. 14). The second strategy addresses "health promotion and disease prevention" and includes "community development." The third is to integrate and coordinate services, and it is here that health districts are introduced as "new organizational arrangements...to help communities work together to achieve the goals of a community-based health system" (1992b, p. 14–16).

The most significant actor to appear in the text of the 1992 documents is a vague, generic, and homogenizing "we." Rather than "I," "you," "us," and "them," the documents are peppered with references to "we," "together," "our," and "Saskatchewan people." Saskatchewan publics and communities are called on to act together and reform health care: "Each of us can take a part in this exciting new venture in health"; and "communities can work toward wellness by tailoring health services to meet local needs" (1992a, p. 4). The new approach will "create a health system that is responsive to community needs by placing control and management responsibilities at a local level" (1992b, p. 11). Also, health reform "is dedicated to encouraging communities and people to actively participate in planning and decision-making" (1992b, p. 14). "After all, mutual aid, partnerships and co-operation are 'the Saskatchewan way' of getting things done" (1992b, p. 24).

After the "we" of Saskatchewan people and communities, the next actor called on in these documents is the government itself (through the Ministry of Health). "Communities and health boards will show leadership at the local level by integrating and delivering services under their own control through health districts" (1992c, p. 6), while the province attends to public policy and supports health districts.

There are occasional references to community representatives, community leaders, health organizations, health professionals and providers, and health care consumers. This new approach to wellness should "involve the general public, community representatives and health professionals as partners with government in the planning, governing and delivery of health programs" (1992b, p. 10). And "we must increase the meaningful involvement and participation of health consumers, communities, and health professionals in the planning, delivery, and governing of health services while respecting the diversity of our population" (1992b, p. 12).

"We," the public, appear in the foreground of this text, while the health system itself (its services, technologies, providers, sites of care, and so forth) appear as background. What is explicit in these texts is that "we," the public, will be involved. "We" are to work in tandem with other people—communities, providers, governments, and organizations—to accomplish a variety of acts. What is less specific in the reports are the actual details and operations of this new model and this new system of health care.

District health boards are introduced as a new organizational structure that will help communities work together to achieve the goals of a community-based health system. "As communities come together to identify their local health needs, they can form a health district and make appropriate decisions regarding the planning, governing and delivery of health services that meet their needs" (1992b, p. 16). Furthermore, "...communities will be encouraged to work together to form health districts, and they will be given the authority to plan, govern and deliver health services that meet shared provincial standards" (1992c, p. 6).

The reports specify that district health boards are organizations that "we" will form and that these organizations will then work towards the goal of health reform and the introduction of a new model of health care, orientated towards community-controlled and community-based wellness. District health boards will determine needs; integrate, coordinate, and manage services (as per provincial guidelines and standards); develop health centres; determine funding allocations (as per needs and core services requirements); make change based on community values; and develop a system that places health decisions in the hands of Saskatchewan people.

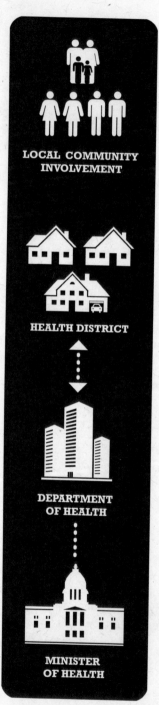

LOCAL COMMUNITY
INVOLVEMENT

HEALTH DISTRICT

DEPARTMENT
OF HEALTH

MINISTER
OF HEALTH

FIGURE 1. THE 1992 MODEL

A flow chart that appears in the 1992 texts (Saskatchewan Health, 1992b, p. 16) is recreated here (see Figure 1). It is interesting in its positioning of "local community involvement" at the top of a chain of action. Although there is no specific line drawn to link the community with any other entry in the diagram, it appears as though it is to work with the newly created districts, which, in turn, work with the Department of Health, which, in turn, works with the Minister of Health.

In general, the three 1992 texts are written for a general, public audience. They are short documents using non-technical language and short, easy sentences. They are about communities and the government, and the new working relationships that will exist between them, via health districts and boards, in the delivering of health services and the governing of the health system. They are active documents, laden with verbs, calling for somewhat generic and vague actions. The texts are grounded in "we," as writer and reader align into a community and collective ethic. In contrast to a more distanced writing style that refers to actions happening "out there" and by "others," this set of texts writes of actions that will happen "here" and by "us."

The 1992 texts resonate with population health logics of public participation and community engagement as routes to empowerment and local control over decisions, and call on political rights and capacities of citizens and communities to participate in local health system governance. They cite consensus, community willingness, and interest as partial reasons for the proposed changes. Publics and communities are inserted into the new governance model with decision-making capacities—not simply as providers of input.

Their partner is portrayed as a government willing to cede and share decision-making control. There is little mention made of the roles of traditional decision makers (for example, providers, managers, etc.), and there is little evidence that consideration was given to the heterogeneous nature of communities, and the particular needs of busy, uninterested, and marginalized community members. The texts assume public participants with necessary interest, time, and knowledge (to plan, govern, assess need, reorient services, and so forth), and paint a somewhat romantic version of egalitarian communities, able to tap into the knowledge and resources within the community and to work together for the health interests of everyone.

THE 2001 ANNOUNCEMENT

After Fyke submitted his 2001 commission report, and before issuing its response to his report, the government completed a round of its own hearings through the Standing Committee on Health. The formal text articulating its strategies and amendments is *The Action Plan for Saskatchewan Health Care* (Saskatchewan Health, 2001). It is a 74-page (double the combined pages of the 1992 texts), letter-size document, written for the Saskatchewan public (although this readership will be commented on below). Premier Lorne Calvert and his Minister of Health, John Nilson, released the report on December 5, 2001. Its precise circulation details are not known.

The inside cover highlights its key actions. Included among these are the establishment of primary health care teams; the introduction of a 24-hour health advice phone line; the adoption of a provincial hospital system ranging from community, to northern, to district, to regional, and to provincial hospitals; and funding for wait-list reductions, health care provider training, a quality council, and health and health services research. The seventh key action is to "reduce administration and improve planning with the formation of 12 Regional Health Authorities to replace 32 districts." This step is then detailed in a six-page chapter entitled "The Plan for the Regional Health Authorities," appearing after chapters that detail plans for primary health care; healthy communities; northern and Aboriginal health; emergency, hospital, and long-term care; wait-lists; providers; and quality care. It is followed by a chapter on sustaining medicare and then closes with two appendices.

One of the earliest shifts in the written text noted when comparing it to the 1992 publications is the site of action or the primary actor. Where the 1992 reports made heavy use of a generic and homogenizing "we," the 2001 report primarily locates its action within specified groups. In particular, it calls on the government, the ministry, and the providers, managers, and administrators of the system. The people of Saskatchewan who were so heavily called upon in the 1992 texts now appear as background, emerging only occasionally, and then primarily as patients and benefactors of these plans as opposed to activists helping to plan and shape the system. Saskatchewan communities appear on occasion in the 2001 text, but again not as primary actors and drivers of reform, but rather as sources of input into, and benefactors of, health system planning. We see a shift from very active and prioritized local involvement and leadership by communities and citizens towards a support role and a service recipient role. The leaders in the 2001 process appear to be the more traditional health system experts, namely the health system managers and administrators, workers, governments, and Regional Health Authorities (appointed by the government). The leaders are no longer the communities and publics (or even their partially elected boards).

Another change readily noted when comparing the 1992 and 2001 texts is the identity of the unnamed reader. While the 1992 reports read as though they were written primarily for the general publics of Saskatchewan, the 2001 text is much longer and more detailed. This might suggest that it was written not only for Saskatchewan publics, but also (and possibly even more so) for the health care workers, providers, managers, and administrators affected by these announced changes and tasked with working in new ways. Where the 1992 reports appeared to be inviting the public in, to work with the system, the 2001 report can be read not so much as an invitation to publics to join in, but rather as a rationale to readers for the plans. Perhaps this is to calm publics and allay concerns after the political backlash the government endured after its 1992 reforms. Perhaps it is to demonstrate the reasoning of the plan and to encourage support through its detail, logic, and rationality, as opposed to encouraging support, as the 1992 texts did, through reference to collective, community, and cooperative spirits.

As with the change in primary actors, the primary actions also change. The 2001 text details more specific actions and events (as opposed to the 1992 texts which described largely unspecified actions). With its specificity and detail, the 2001 text casts an ethos of rationality, efficiency, and effectiveness, with planned transitions led by experts, where the 1992 text can be read to call on communitarian traditions and cooperative ethics.

Where "we" would form the district health boards (or so the 1992 text implied) to achieve the goals of health reform, and where boards were written of as working for local communities, the Regional Health Authorities (RHAS) were to be formed by the government and were positioned as managerial and administrative structures more than community engagement sites. Community linkage in the RHA model is to occur through a new structure, the Community Advisory Network (CAN). This relocating of community engagement goals and activities to the Community Advisory Networks—as opposed to within the Regional Health Authorities themselves, even though the RHAS are boards comprised of community members—marks a significant shift in the discourse and one that has received impressively little critical consideration in studies of regionalization.

Not only has the primary site of direct community involvement been moved out one step, but so, too, have community members' roles. Community involvement is emphasized less in this 2001 iteration and is retracted to the provision of input to and communication with Regional Health Authorities. It is not clear the extent to which this is an intentional shift in language, but it does reposition boards more as administrative structures and less as active, political, and democratic structures, while locating public participation (through Community Advisory Networks) towards the technocratic end of an artificial—and, admittedly, an overly simplistic—technocratic-democratic public participation continuum.

Another contrast between the texts appears when we consider the diagram that appeared in the 1992 text (see Figure 1). As noted in the previous section, community appeared at the top of this diagram and, indeed, the tone and language of the texts implied that communities would drive the action. The 2001 text can be read as inverting this flow so that the government and its health department lead in working with the Regional Health Authorities, which then involve and communicate with "the community" via their Community Advisory Network. The original 1992 flow chart would then be inverted (see Figure 2).

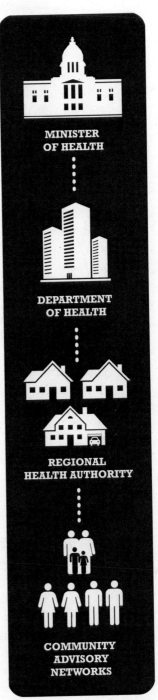

MINISTER
OF HEALTH

DEPARTMENT
OF HEALTH

REGIONAL
HEALTH AUTHORITY

COMMUNITY
ADVISORY
NETWORKS

FIGURE 2. THE 2001 MODEL

Although the 2001 amendments appear to value linkage between citizens and the health system through the Community Advisory Networks, and by having community members serve as appointed governors of their regional authority, gone are the explicit references so visible in the 1992 announcements linking regionalization to citizen engagement, public participation, community involvement and decision-making, communities as partners with local control and accountability, and other markers of population health and democratic logics.

The 2001 text calls instead on technocratic logics that favour rationality, expertise, and centralized planning. Publics are called on, but in more restricted capacities, as individuals and patients with input and advice to offer to others who actually plan and make decisions. Local elections will no longer be used to elect a portion of the boards; instead, government appointments will constitute entire boards. While perhaps correcting for the overly romantic visions of community painted in the 1992 texts, the 2001 text inverts the earlier model to call instead on more technocratic notions of decision-making and system governance; there is no mention of population health strategies of engagement and empowerment, nor of the political rights and capacities of citizens and communities to participate. In these ways, the 2001 text appears to prioritize experts and traditional decision makers—with necessary interest, time, and knowledge to plan, govern, assess need, and reorient services—over publics and communities.

CONCLUSIONS

Both the 1992 and 2001 models of regionalization and public participation represented in these texts carry with them problematic assumptions. They assume (the 1992 texts more so) that communities and publics are ready, interested, and available to assume new roles and duties as governors, responsible citizens, volunteers, workers, providers of input, or even ad hoc advisors. The validity of this assumption has been questioned (e.g., Side & Keefe, 2004), and the tendency of health reforms to shift health system work to unpaid sites has been detailed (e.g., Armstrong et al., 2001).

Both sets of texts also assume that these new roles and new spaces are open to and relevant for all. Even when comprised of appointed members (as opposed to those elected), data has shown that health boards overrepresent traditionally privileged groups, while failing to represent the general Canadian population (Chessie, 2009; Lomas, Veenstra, & Woods, 1997b; Lewis et al., 2001).

Neither do the 1992 or 2001 texts account for research showing that traditional participation avenues, such as boards, public meetings, and focus groups or surveys, marginalize many publics (Wharf Higgins, 1999), and that "one-size-fits-all" models do not work for all communities and publics. As Abelson (2001) noted, different communities have different participation styles that vary along class, cultural, and religious lines. We must appreciate these differences. This assumption is problematic for the 2001 text, which valued centralization and sought to reduce intraprovincial variability. The 1992 texts allowed for local variation, but then assumed homogeneous communities that would bring knowledge of the health needs and resources to the table, and that would be ready, willing, and able to work together for everyone's interests.

Consider again the varying continuums along which public participation has been theorized, with participation rooted in the abilities of publics to: contribute knowledge (via experiential and/or credentialed expertise) and legitimacy (via democratic rights); participate as individuals or as representatives of groups, as experts, patients, taxpayers, or citizens; contribute to micro-level service planning up through to macro-level issues of governance and policy; fill roles ranging from passive receipt of information to provision of input to active shared decision-making and power (Arnstein, 1969; Charles & DeMaio, 1993; Collins & Evans, 2002; Tritter & McCallum, 2006). In this paper, these roles and positions have been further organized into those supported by logics of population health, democratic legitimacy, and accountability, or those supported by logics of technocratic decision-making advantage.

Under both the 1992 and 2001 models, public participation in health system decision-making and governance lacks a necessary clarity around the precise nature of that public involvement. This was particularly evident in the 1992 model. Its introductory texts were rooted in communitarian-like ethics that opened wide the field of health system governance to public participation and control. While this may have offered the potential to empower and bring legitimacy to health reform strategies and governance—and was thus plausibly linked to democratic and population health gains—this participation came at the expense of the equally legitimate and necessary contributions of experts, and without visible consideration of the real and necessary limits to community capacities. We then see a retraction in this positioning of publics with the 2001 text, as the discourse shifts and technical expertise is reinserted. However, this comes at the expense of plausible legitimacy gains offered through widened community and public participation, and potential population health gains rooted in community engagement and empowerment.

We need to appreciate the distinctions in roles and supporting logics of public participation in health system policy and governance, and we need to consider their implications when theorizing and establishing public participation models. Publicly funded services such as health care are about more than technical issues and considerations. Publicly funded health care is at least in part about social ethics and the redistribution of privilege and resources from wealthier, healthier citizens to those with less, and in this way can be tied to collective considerations of what is best for everyone. We can lose sight of these collective ends when we attend only to our individualized, client- and patient-level concerns and experiences with health care and service delivery. As citizens, publics have political rights that buoy involvement in health care governance and policy deliberations, and their participation has the potential to contribute to better and more legitimate decisions. Democratic considerations aside, participating in and contributing to the decisions that affect our lives have also been tied to population health gains (Epp, 1986; WHO, 1986). With these two logics, public participation is a necessary—but not sufficient—condition for good decision-making. Health service elites (for example, care providers, managers, policy researchers, and decision makers) also have legitimate and necessary contributions, rooted in their technical knowledge and expertise, which buoy their involvement in the deliberations and decision-making. All three of these routes and logics need to be considered when positing models of public participation.

Neither the 1992 nor the 2001 model considered in this paper fused these logics to posit models of public participation that balanced issues of technical questions and the contributions of expertise with engagement and empowerment logics of population health determinants and with considerations of democratic accountability and legitimacy. We need to articulate models that call on the strengths of each, rather than ignoring roles or pitting citizens against experts, deliberating technical questions of services at the expense of democratic questions of equity, or at the expense of population health exercises of engagement and empowerment. Only in balancing all three logics can we move beyond unduly constrained "either/or" models, to those where citizens, communities, and systems of health all benefit from exercising multiple configurations of participation rights, accountabilities, and expertise. All three logics offer different strengths and potentials worthy of consideration, and public participation models need to become more sophisticated and account for the three simultaneously. In this way, we may maximally benefit from public participation and move to accurate and informed, legitimate and accountable, equitable and healthy decision-making and governance models.

NOTES

1. Public policies of health system regionalization and community involvement were not entirely new: Saskatchewan had endorsed regionalization after Sigerist (1944), and a health region existed in the Swift Current area from the mid-1940s to the 1990s (Feather, 1991; Houston, 2002; Taylor, 1987).

2. Premier Grant Devine and his Conservative government established the Murray Commission in 1988. The commission investigated issues affecting "the quality, availability, accessibility, and cost" of health services, with a "particular consideration of the differences between rural and urban communities." Citing a province in transition (its demography, family structures, illness patterns, service delivery, and costs) it concluded that the system must change with it, while respecting its principles and history. Its recommendations were rooted in an idea that "the people it serves must have the ownership and responsibility for their local health care system, must determine how it is used and managed and establish its priorities" (Murray, 1990, p. 4). It recommended, amongst other things, "a system divided into health service divisions governed by powerful health councils that are locally elected and funded mainly through the Department of Health" (Murray, 1990, p. 4).

3. The December 2001 announcements were made while the Legislative Assembly was not in session and, thus, no Hansard proceedings are available for this period.

4. Romanow had resigned and would eventually appear on the federal scene to lead the Commission on the Future of Health Care.

REFERENCES

Abelson, J. (2001). Understanding the role of contextual influences on local health-care decision making: Case study results from Ontario, Canada. *Social Science and Medicine, 53*, 777–793.

Abelson, J., Forest, P. G., Eyels, J., Smith, P., Martin, E., & Gauvin, F. P. (2003). Deliberation about deliberative methods: Issues in the design and evaluation of public participation processes. *Science & Medicine, 57*, 239–251.

Adams, D. (2001). The white and the black horse race: Saskatchewan health reform in the 1990s. In H. Leeson (Ed.), *Saskatchewan politics into the twenty-first century* (pp. 267–294). Regina: Canadian Plains Research Center.

Armstrong, P., Amaratunga, C., Bernier, J., & Grant, K. (2001). *Exposing privatization: Women and health care reform in Canada*. Aurora, ON: Garamond Press.

Arnstein, S. R. (1969). A ladder of citizen participation in the USA. *Journal of the American Institute of Planners, 35*, 214–224.

Baggott, R. (2005). A funny thing happened on the way to the forum? Reforming patient and public involvement in the NHS and England. *Public Administration, 83*, 533–551.

Charles, C., & DeMaio, S. (1993). Lay participation in health care decision making: A conceptual framework. *Journal of Health Politics, Policy & Law, 18*, 881–904.

Chessie, K. (2009). Health system regionalization in Canada's provincial and territorial health systems: Do citizen governance boards represent, engage and empower? *International Journal of Health Services, 39*, 705–724.

Church, J., Saunders, D., Wanke, M., Pong, R., Spooner, C., & Dorgan, M. (2002). Citizen participation in health decision-making: Past experience and future prospects. *Journal of Public Health Policy, 32*, 12–32.

Clair, M. (2001). *Emerging solutions: Report and recommendations.* Quebec City: Commission d'étude sur les services de santé et les services sociaux.

Collins, H. M., & Evans, R. (2002). The third wave of science studies: Studies of expertise and experience. *Social Studies of Science, 32,* 235–296.

Crichton, A., Robertson, A., Gordon, C., & Farrant, W. (1997). *Health care: A community concern?* Calgary: University of Calgary Press.

Davies, C., Wetherell, M., & Barnett, E. (2006). *Citizens at the centre: Deliberative participation in health care decisions.* Bristol: The Policy Press.

Deber, R. (1996). International experiences with decentralization and regionalization: Northern Europe. In J. Dorland & M. S. Davis (Eds.), *How many roads? Regionalization and decentralization in health care* (pp. 53–62). Queen's CMA Conference on Regionalization & Decentralization in Health Care. Kingston: Queen's School of Policy Studies.

Dickinson, H. D. (2004). Public involvement in the development of a health care vision. In P.-G. Forest, G. P. Marchildon, & T. McIntosh (Eds.), *Changing health care in Canada: The Romanow papers, volume 2* (pp. 243–278). Toronto: University of Toronto.

Drache, D., & Sullivan, T. (1999). Health reform and market talk: Rhetoric and reality. In D. Drache & T. Sullivan, (Eds.), *Market limits in health reform: Public success, private failure* (pp. 1–22). London: Routledge.

Dwyer, J. (2004). Regionalization: Are even the flaws quintessentially Canadian? *Healthcare Papers, 5,* 81–87.

Epp, J. (1986). *Achieving health for all: A framework for health promotion.* Ottawa, ON: Health and Welfare Canada.

Fairclough, N. (1989). *Language and power.* London: Longman Press.

Feather, J. (1991). Impact of the Swift Current Health Region: Experiment or model? *Prairie Forum, 16*(2), 225–248.

Frankish, J., Kwan, B., Ratner, P. A., & Wharf Higgins, J. (1999). *Community participation in health-system decision making.* Survey 3 in a Series of Surveys of Health Authorities in British Columbia. Vancouver: Institute of Health Promotion Research, UBC.

Fyke, K. (2001). *Caring for medicare: Sustaining a quality system.* (Final Report of the Saskatchewan Commission on Medicare). Regina: The Commission.

Government of Ontario. (2006). *Local Health System Integration Act, 2006.* S.O. 2006, Chapter 4.

Gray, J., Delaquis, S., & Closson, T. (2008). *Report of the Manitoba Regional Health Authority External Review Committee.* Winnipeg: Government of Manitoba.

Hansen, P. (2003). *Taxing illusions: Taxation, democracy and embedded political theory.* Halifax: Fernwood Publishing.

Houston, C. S. (2002). *Steps on the road to medicare: Why Saskatchewan led the way.* Montreal: McGill-Queen's University Press.

Hyndman, L. (chair). (1989). *The Rainbow Report: Our vision for health.* Edmonton, AB: Premier's Commission on Future of Health Care for Albertans.

Kouri, D., Chessie, K., & Lewis, S. (2002). *Regionalization: Where has all the power gone? A survey of Canadian decision-makers in health care regionalization.* Saskatoon: Canadian Centre for the Analysis of Regionalization and Health.

Legislative Assembly of Saskatchewan (1992a). Debates and Proceedings (Hansard) of the Legislative Assembly of Saskatchewan. July 17, 1992, to September 17, 1992. Accessed June 2008 from http://www.legassembly.sk.ca/Hansard/hansard92.htm

Legislative Assembly of Saskatchewan (1992b). Debates and Proceedings (Hansard) of the Legislative Assembly of Saskatchewan. April 27, 1992. Downloaded June 10, 2008, from http://www.legassembly.sk.ca/Hansard/hansard92.htm

Legislative Assembly of Saskatchewan (1993). Debates and Proceedings (Hansard) of the Legislative Assembly of Saskatchewan. February 25, 1993. Downloaded June 10, 2008, from http://www.legassembly.sk.ca/Hansard/hansard92.htm

Legislative Assembly of Saskatchewan (2001). Debates and Proceedings (Hansard) of the Legislative Assembly of Saskatchewan. March 20, 2001. Downloaded June 10, 2008, from http://www.legassembly.sk.ca/Hansard/hansard2001.htm

Legislative Assembly of Saskatchewan (2002). Debates and Proceedings (Hansard) of the Legislative Assembly of Saskatchewan. March 14, 2002. Downloaded June 10, 2008, from http://www.legassembly.sk.ca/Hansard/hansard2001.htm

Lewis, S. (1997). Regionalization and devolution: Transforming health, reshaping politics? Occasional Paper No. 2. Saskatoon: HEALNet Regional Health Planning.

Lewis, S., Kouri, D., Estabrooks, C. A., Dickinson, H., Dutchak, J. J., Williams, J. I., Mustard, C., & Hurley, J. (2001). Devolution to democratic health authorities in Saskatchewan: An interim report. Canadian Medical Association Journal, 164(3), 343–347.

Liepert, R. (2008). Minister's open letter to Albertans. May 15, 2008. Downloaded June 10, 2008, from http://www.health.alberta.ca/regions/HSB_Open-letter.html

Lomas, J. (1996). Devolved authorities in Canada: The new sites of health-care system conflict? In J. Dorland and M. S. Davis (Eds.), How many roads? Regionalization and decentralization in health care (pp. 3–10). Queen's CMA Conference on Regionalization & Decentralization in Health Care. Kingston: Queen's School of Policy Studies.

Lomas, J. (1999). The evolution of devolution: what does the community want? In D. Drache & T. Sullivan (Eds.), Market limits in health reform: Public success, private failure (pp. 166–185). London: Routledge.

Lomas, J., Veenstra, G., & Woods, J. (1997a). Devolving authority for health care in Canada's provinces: 2. Backgrounds, resources and activities of board members. Canadian Medical Association Journal, 156(4), 513–520.

Lomas, J., Veenstra, G., & Woods, J. (1997b). Devolving authority for health care in Canada's provinces: 3. Motivations, attitudes and approaches of board members. Canadian Medical Association Journal, 156(5), 669–676.

Lomas, J., Woods, J., & Veenstra, G. (1997). Devolving authority for health care in Canada's provinces: 1. An introduction to the issues. Canadian Medical Association Journal, 156(3), 371–377.

MacKinnon, M. P. (2006). Citizens: An underused and undervalued asset in the pursuit of improved health care delivery. Ottawa: Canadian Policy Research Networks.

Marchildon, G. P. (2005). Health systems in transition: Canada. Copenhagen: WHO Regional Office for Europe on behalf of the European Observatory on Health Systems and Policies.

Mazankowski, D. (2001). A framework for reform. Report of the Premier's Advisory Council on Health. Edmonton, AB: Premier's Advisory Council on Health for Alberta.

McIntosh, T., & Marchildon, G. P. (Forthcoming). The Fyke in the road: Health reform in Saskatchewan from Romanow to Calvert and beyond.

Mhatre, S. L., & Deber, R. B. (1992). From equal access to health care to equitable access to health: A review of Canadian provincial health commissions and reports. International Journal of Health Services, 22, 645–68.

Morgan, L. (2001). Community participation in health: Persistent allure, persistent challenge. Health Policy & Planning, 16(3), 221–230.

Murray, R. G. (1990). *Future directions for health care in Saskatchewan*. Report of the Saskatchewan Commission on Directions in Health Care.

New Brunswick. (2008). *Transforming New Brunswick's health-care system: The Provincial Health Plan 2008–2012*. Fredericton: Province of New Brunswick.

Nova Scotia Commission on Health Care. (1989). *The report of the Nova Scotia Commission on Health Care: Towards a new strategy: Summary*. Halifax: Nova Scotia Commission on Health Care.

Prince Edward Island Ministry of Health. (2006). *Ministry of Health annual report 2005–2006*. Charlottetown: Government of Prince Edward Island.

Rasmussen, K. (2001). Regionalization and collaborative government: A new direction for health system governance. In D. Adams (Ed.), *Federalism, democracy and health policy in Canada* (pp. 239–270). Kingston: Queen's University Press.

Rochon, J. (Chair). (1987). *Rapport de la Commission d'Enquête sur les Services de Santé et les Services Sociaux*. Quebec: Government of Quebec.

Rogers, R. (2004). *An introduction to critical discourse analysis in education*. New Jersey: Lawrence Erlbaum Associates Publishers.

Saskatchewan Health. (1992a). *A Saskatchewan vision for health*. Regina, SK: Government of Saskatchewan.

Saskatchewan Health. (1992b). *A Saskatchewan vision for health: A framework for change*. Regina, SK: Government of Saskatchewan.

Saskatchewan Health. (1992c). *A Saskatchewan vision for health: Challenges and opportunities*. Regina, SK: Government of Saskatchewan.

Saskatchewan Health. (2001). *Healthy people, a healthy province: The action plan for Saskatchewan health care*. Regina, SK: Government of Saskatchewan.

Scutchfield, F. D., Ireson, C., & Hall, L. (2004). The voice of the public in public health policy and planning. *Journal of Health Policy, 25*, 197–205.

Seaton, P. (Chair) (1991). *Closer to home: Report of the British Columbia Royal Commission on health care and costs*. Victoria, BC: British Columbia Royal Commission on Health Care and Costs.

Side, K., & Keefe, J. (2004). Health regionalization and rurality in Nova Scotia. *Canadian Review of Social Policy, 54*, 108–116.

Sigerist, H. (1944). *Report of the Commissioner for the Saskatchewan Health Services Survey Commission*. Regina: King's Printer.

Smith, D. (1990). *Texts, facts, and femininity: Exploring the relations of ruling*. Routledge: London.

Taylor, M. G. (1987). *Health insurance and Canadian public policy: The seven decisions that created the Canadian Health Insurance System*. Montreal: McGill-Queen's University Press.

Taylor, J., Wilkinson, D., & Cheers, B. (2006). Is it consumer or community participation? Examining the links between "community" and "participation." *Health Sociology Review, 15*, 38–47.

Tritter, J., & McCallum, A. (2006). The snakes and ladders of user involvement: Moving beyond Arnstein. *Health Policy, 76*, 156–168.

Veenstra, G., & Lomas, J. (1999). Home is where the governing is: Social capital and regional health governance. *Health & Place, 5*, 1–12.

Wetzel, K. (2005). *Labour relations and health reform: A comparative study of five jurisdictions*. New York: Palgrave McMillan.

Wharf Higgins, J. (1999). Closer to home: The case for experiential participation in health reform. *Canadian Journal of Public Health, 90*, 30–4.

World Health Organization. (1986). *Ottawa Charter for health promotion*. Ottawa, ON.

Wodak, R., & Meyer, M. (2001). *Methods of critical discourse analysis*. London: Sage.

"A Healthy Pregnancy is in Your Hands": Agency, Regulation, and the Importance of Social Difference to Women's Experiences of the Medicalization of Pregnancy

Janelle Hippe

Once understood as a normal and natural process, today pregnancy has been redefined by medical experts as a time full of potential dangers, and pregnant women have become the subject of a vast array of expert knowledge and interventions purportedly designed to monitor and eliminate any risks to a healthy pregnancy outcome (Barker, 1998; Mitchinson, 1998; 2002; Oakley, 1984). On the surface of it, this "medicalization" (Zola, 1972) of pregnancy may be understood as a positive phenomenon that increases pregnant women's health information and options. It is in this vein, for example, that the Public Health Agency of Canada's (PHAC) "Healthy Pregnancy" campaign advises women: "A Healthy Pregnancy is in your Hands." According to the PHAC's *Sensible Guide to a Healthy Pregnancy*, women can increase their agency in the pregnancy process by utilizing the expert knowledge offered by medical researchers, epidemiologists, nutritionists, and doctors to make the best possible choices regarding tobacco, alcohol, nutrition, folic acid, and oral health (PHAC, 2008).

Yet, while the proliferation of medical expertise surrounding pregnancy may increase women's health information and options, the medicalization of pregnancy can have negative consequences as well. For example, public health messages that highlight the importance of adherence to expert medical advice can draw attention away from social factors that can significantly affect pregnancy outcomes, such as abuse, social support, and income adequacy

(Feldman et al., 2000; Kramer et al., 2000; Muhajarine & D'Arcy, 1999; Campbell, 2001; Murphy et al., 2001). Because the medicalization of pregnancy can operate to push to the background the social factors that affect pregnancy outcomes, women's agency can be reduced—or regulated—in the sense that all women are tacitly compelled to follow expert advice and implicitly blamed if they experience adverse pregnancy outcomes (Morgan, 1998; Oaks, 2000; Ruhl, 1999).

The negative consequences of medicalization may be particularly acute for women who have been identified as "at risk" of adverse pregnancy outcomes. Many health researchers have begun to argue, for example, that the epidemiological identification of "risk groups" can contribute to negative stereotypes of individuals within these groups as lacking the willpower or moral integrity to adhere to expert knowledge (Brown & Smye, 2002; McDermott, 1998; O'Neil, Reading, & Leader, 1998; Poudrier, 2007). Such negative stereotypes, in turn, can function as an implicit justification for intensified surveillance (Shim, 2000; O'Neil, Reading, & Leader, 1998).

In Canada, epidemiological evidence suggests that adverse pregnancy outcomes are statistically highest among young women, poor women, and Aboriginal women (Dyck et al., 2002; Kramer et al., 2000; Luo et al., 2004; PHAC, 2000; Wenman, Joffres, & Tataryn, 2004). As such, there are reasons to suspect that social differences such as age, income level, and Aboriginal-/non-Aboriginal identity may affect the extent of agency or regulation that pregnant women experience in relation to expert knowledge. However, there is little Canadian research that has explored how these social differences can affect women's experiences of the medicalization of their pregnancies.

This paper thus presents and theoretically contextualizes the results of qualitative research that was designed to understand how social differences such as age, Aboriginal/non-Aboriginal identity, and income level can affect pregnant women's experiences of the medicalization of pregnancy. In the following section of this paper, I review theoretical material that addresses the relationship between expertise and agency (Giddens, 1990; 1999; Foucault, 1976; 1990; 1995). Subsequent to this, I present and discuss the results of interviews conducted with 10 Aboriginal and 10 non-Aboriginal women of varying ages and income levels during their pregnancies. Specifically, the results presented in this paper address: (1) How social differences, such as age, Aboriginal/non-Aboriginal identity, and income affect women's experiences with expert knowledge; and (2) How such social differences affect women's experiences with health experts.

AGENCY, REGULATION, AND EXPERTISE: KEY SOCIOLOGICAL CONCEPTS

The large body of sociological literature that has grown to address the modern rise of both medical and non-medical expertise offers at least two alternate ways of theorizing the impact of medicalization on pregnant women's agency. First, there are frameworks that stress the modern individual's capacity for reflexivity (Beck, 1999; Williams & Calnan, 1996; Giddens, 1990; 1999). This framework has been particularly well developed in the work of Anthony Giddens.

For Giddens, it is our modern ability to communicate and form social relationships that stretch across time and space that has facilitated the rise of far-reaching and more or less standardized "expert" systems of knowledge, such as modern systems of medicine or law (Giddens, 1990). While these expert systems of knowledge are essentially ubiquitous and inescapable, expert knowledge is also highly specialized. As such, lay individuals have no direct access to this knowledge, but instead must depend on "system representatives," such as doctors or lawyers, to simplify and communicate this knowledge to them (Giddens, 1990, p. 85). At the same time, Giddens notes that the knowledge produced by experts can be contradictory and is always changing. This can create a potentially confusing and helpless situation for the modern individual, who is subject to a continually changing pool of knowledge that she can never fully understand. Yet for Giddens, the modern individual is neither confused nor helpless in the face of expert knowledge because she is characteristically reflexive: the modern individual is able to thoughtfully evaluate both the contents of expert knowledge claims and "system representatives" themselves (Giddens, 1990; Williams & Calnan, 1996).

Significantly, Giddens' work is also underlain by the notion that expert knowledge is essentially progressive to the extent that it is freed from the constraints of "tradition" (Peterson, 1996; Giddens, 1999). Together, the key concepts of progress and reflexivity suggest that the expansion of expert knowledge surrounding pregnancy increases women's agency because it expands the information and choices available to them. This suggests that the importance of social difference to women's experiences of medicalization relates to the different social constraints women may experience as they attempt to access and utilize expert knowledge.

An alternate framework for theorizing the rise of expert knowledge is developed in the work of Michel Foucault (Foucault, 1995; 1990; 1976). According to a Foucauldian analysis, modern systems of scientific knowledge do not enhance individual agency; they regulate it. For Foucault, the rise of expert knowledge is propelled by a modern shift in the focus of governance—from controlling a territory to regulating a population (1976). Modern expertise, such as that produced in demography or medicine, is characterized, for Foucault, by a panoptic surveillance of the population and all the individuals within it (1995; 1990). Empirical manifestations of this panoptic surveillance include the statistics about birth rates and death rates produced by demographers as well as the medical and epidemiological surveillance that produces knowledge about health, illness, and statistical "risks" to well-being (Foucault, 1990, p. 171). This surveillance of the population regulates individuals through producing knowledge about what is normal and pathological—"risky" and safe—and enacting a power that works through people as they attempt to conform to the norm (Foucault, 1990; Armstrong, 1995; Shim, 2000; Rose, 1993; Rose & Miller, 1992). Indeed, for Foucault, expert knowledge generates not only conformity, but also identity, as individuals are invited to understand themselves through the labels—*healthy* and *ill*; *risky* and *safe*; *normal* and *pathological*—that are created through production of expert knowledge.

Foucault's key insights surrounding surveillance, identity, and conformity suggest that knowledge is always inextricably linked to the power that labels and regulates us. In this analysis of expert knowledge, the medicalization of pregnancy is accompanied by the construction of "normal" and "pathological" identities and "normal" and "pathological" behaviours. At the same time, the concept of reflexive agency is replaced by the concept of regulated agency, as women are compelled to conform to expert rules while the social structural causes of health differentials are obscured. The importance of social difference, in such a framework, extends beyond women's ability to access and utilize expert knowledge; rather, Foucault's framework suggests that social difference may be important to women's experiences of pathologization and regulation, since different women may be differentially labelled, monitored, and controlled.

METHODS

In order to explore how social differences such as Aboriginal/non-Aboriginal identity, age, and income affect women's experiences with medical expertise, I sought to include both Aboriginal and non-Aboriginal women from varying income levels and age groups during their pregnancies. To recruit my sample, I employed a modified form of Arcury and Quandt's (1999) site-based approach to participant recruitment. This involved contacting and arranging meetings with individuals in directorial positions—or "gatekeepers"—at community centres or community-oriented services for women with children. At these meetings I explained the nature of my study and the demographic that I wished to interview. I brought several recruitment letters to each meeting and asked the gatekeeper to provide a copy of the letter to women who indicated interest in partaking in the study. The recruitment letter contained a brief description of the study and details about what was required of participants, along with my contact information. In one case, the gatekeeper thought it would be more suitable to explain the study to women she thought might be interested and provide me with a copy of the phone numbers of women who indicated they would like to participate. When women contacted me about the study, or, in the latter case, when I contacted women who indicated their interest in participating, I explained the details of the study once more before confirming their interest in participating. I then set up a time and date that was mutually convenient to do the interview.

The participants of this study included 10 Aboriginal and 10 non-Aboriginal[1] women who were or had been pregnant. Among the Aboriginal women I interviewed, household incomes during pregnancy ranged from social assistance to $100,000/year. Among the non-Aboriginal women I interviewed, household incomes during pregnancy ranged from social assistance to $95,000/year. Six of the 10 non-Aboriginal women I interviewed lived in a household with an income near or below the poverty line[2] for at least one of their pregnancies. Seven of the 10 Aboriginal women I interviewed lived in a household with an income near or below the poverty line during at least one of their pregnancies. Of the 20 women that I interviewed, 12 were pregnant during their teenage years. Four of the non-Aboriginal women had been pregnant as teenagers and eight of the Aboriginal women had children as teenagers.

The interview schedule was semi-structured and divided into six sections that included questions designed to:

1) orient women to the topic;

2) address women's experiences with prenatal programs, health care workers, and doctors;

3) address women's feelings of control as they interacted with health experts;

4) address women's sources of knowledge as well as their opinions about "expert" knowledge;

5) address the idea of "risk" and the social-structural health challenges that women faced during their pregnancies;

6) address age, "race," income, and experiences of discrimination during pregnancy.

At the end of the interview I collected socio-demographic information that had not come up during the course of the interview. The average interview length was one and a half hours. Each participant signed a consent form before the interviews and was given a twenty-dollar unadvertised honorarium after the interview. Interviews were tape-recorded and transcribed verbatim. The names of the women, their children, doctors, and any other identifying information were changed to ensure the anonymity of the women interviewed.

My aim during coding and analysis of the interviews was to discern both what different women have in common and what experiences are particular to specific groups of women as women experience, internalize, and interact with experts and expert knowledge during pregnancy. Drawing on directives laid out by Miles and Huberman (1994) and Lofland and Lofland (1995), I addressed these questions through the development of both theoretical and grounded codes. Theoretical codes drew on the framework summarized in the previous section. Thus, drawing on both Foucault and Giddens, I developed theoretical codes to highlight instances of regulation and individualization, as well as instances of agency or reflexivity. Grounded codes were used to highlight issues that arose as important to the topic of analysis, but that were not previously considered in the theoretical framework.

RESULTS

Social Difference and Women's Experiences with Expert Knowledge

In my interviews with women about their experiences during their pregnancies, all women tended to feel that "expert" knowledge surrounding pregnancy was important and all women tended to solicit expert knowledge from a variety of sources, including prenatal programs, doctors, books, and the Internet. Across social differences, gathering "expert" knowledge about pregnancy made women feel more educated and more "prepared" for both pregnancy and labour. At the same time, many participants indicated to me that they also drew on mothers, family, or friends to solicit knowledge about pregnancy. Indeed, women frequently expressed the idea that "expertise" surrounding pregnancy was something that required a blend of both medical and experiential knowledge. However, in instances where women compared the value and legitimacy of expert versus experiential knowledge, many women considered knowledge gleaned from "expert" sources to have a "scientific" legitimacy that experiential knowledge did not. For example, many women indicated to me that if they wanted to know something "for sure," they would ask a doctor or a health professional.

While women felt expert knowledge was important to prepare, and while expert knowledge emerged as having a "scientific" legitimacy that experiential knowledge did not, many women also linked expert knowledge to control. For example, when I asked Marie why she participated in a prenatal program, she replied: "Just so I could get all the benefits I could find. Learn as much as I could. If a person is educated as much as they can be...they make fewer mistakes." Jesse, on the other hand, identified the nutritional knowledge she gained from a book as particularly helpful:

> With my pregnancy...the book helped a lot. My first pregnancy... I don't think I would have had the diet that I had when I was pregnant. I don't think I would have had the knowledge...you have too much of this...this is what could happen...or you know...you've got to try and stay away from sugar as much as possible...And to me, that [the book] was my most helpful thing.

Across social differences, women made such links between the appropriation of expert knowledge and the control to "make fewer mistakes." Together with the fact that most women solicited knowledge from both expert and non-expert sources, such as friends or mothers, these results suggest that the proliferation of expert knowledge surrounding pregnancy works across social differences to give women more health information and options, more choices, and thus, more agency in relation to their own and their baby's health. However, when the interviews turned to the topic of risk and responsibility, links between expert knowledge and control could underlie a process of individualization in which women felt that they alone bore the main responsibility for their baby's health.

When I asked women what the phrase "health risk" made them think of or what they felt were the main "risks" to healthy pregnancies, women's responses tended to fall into three categories. First, some women linked the notion of "risk" to prior health conditions that could constitute a "risk" to a healthy pregnancy, such as diabetes or obesity. Second, women who had been in abusive relationships during their pregnancies tended to cite these relationships as "risks" to healthy pregnancies. Third, most frequently, and with no obvious relationship to social difference, women's responses about the main "risks" to healthy pregnancies tended to echo "expert" knowledge surrounding smoking, drinking, or using drugs during pregnancy. Frequent associations between "risk" and behaviour also tended to be intertwined with the notion that many of the "risks" to health during pregnancy are controllable. For example, when I asked LeAnn what the phrase "health risk" made her think of in relation to pregnancy, she replied: "Well...when I think health risk I do think of things like...smoking...things like...lifestyle choices...do you drink alcohol, do you do drugs…those kinds of things are what I think of when I think of risk." For Christine, the kinds of things that put women's health at risk during their pregnancies were choices:

> You choose to put on your seat belt or you don't. You choose to… you know…have…drugs or whatever…or have a cigarette or go and have that one glass of wine…[…] Health risks are anything that you could do or you don't. You choose not to.

While my questions about "risk" frequently suggested that women associated the notion of "health risks" during pregnancy with controllable behavioural "choices," the importance of exercise, vitamins, and nutrition often arose spontaneously throughout the interviews. Ultimately, when I asked women if they felt they had control over their own health and whether or not their baby was born healthy, most of the women I spoke with related to me that they felt that because they could control "how they took care of themselves," they felt they had considerable control over both their own health and whether or not their baby was healthy.

In light of the results discussed above, it is unsurprising that most of the women I spoke with felt that pregnant women bore the main responsibility for their own and their baby's health. In the narratives of some women, the notion that women are responsible for the outcomes of their pregnancies and the notion that women can control these outcomes through adherence to expert knowledge could underlie a sense of guilt or self-blame when women failed to adhere to expert knowledge. For example, Rene recalled the guilt she felt the one time she drank during her most recent pregnancy:

> With Ethan, I drank once. And I felt so guilty. And I think the guilt hurt me more than…that one night of drinking. Oh my god…the next six months, I'm worried that he's going to be Fetal Alcohol Syndrome because I drank one night. And so it's like…causes stress to worry about that…because they're saying you can't even have a glass.

While associations between expert knowledge, responsibility, and control could lead to instances of guilt and self-blame, some participants also levelled negative judgment at other women who were perceived to disregard expert knowledge. For example, when I asked Andrea what she felt were the main risks to a healthy pregnancy, she replied:

I would say…probably drugs and alcohol. If these girls could see what that does to these babies and they're so innocent. They don't ask for that. I mean just because you can't control yourself not having a drink or shooting up and that…why should your child pay for that? Cause they're the ones that pay for it in the long run. So…I don't know. Like if they could see what it does and how these babies suffer from it. You'd hope that it would make them think twice, but half of them don't. How can you hurt your kid that way? I don't know.

The negative judgment that was sometimes levelled at women who were perceived to disregard expert knowledge suggests that links between expert knowledge and control can underlie a process of mutual surveillance, where women monitor and judge not only their own, but also other women's adherence to expert knowledge during pregnancy.

While social differences among women appeared to have little effect on the ways that women interacted with, experienced, or internalized expert knowledge during their pregnancy, age and Aboriginal identity could bear on women's pregnancy experiences when women experienced judgment that was related to the very fact of their being pregnant. Thus, when the interviews turned to the topic of the experience of pregnancy more generally and social views on pregnancy, women who had had children when they were older frequently felt that their pregnancies were viewed positively by many of the people they came into contact with. On the other hand, women who had had children when they were younger often recalled feeling judgment related to the negatively perceived moral character of the young, pregnant woman.

The judgment that women felt when they were young and pregnant was frequently exacerbated for Aboriginal women. For example, when I asked Cathy how "race" and age affect the experience of pregnancy, she replied:

Well let me start by saying this. When I was pregnant, getting on the bus was like one of the hardest things to do. Because you have all these people staring at you. Like…I remember thinking oh god… like all these people think here's another Native girl…who's however old…teenage girl getting pregnant again and I just felt like I was getting looks from people. People would look down on me. Like I'm a bad person or something. Like that I wasn't good enough. […] That's how I felt I was viewed by a lot of people.

Cathy's sense that people were "looking down on her" because she was a young, pregnant Aboriginal woman was by no means imagined. When I asked non-Aboriginal women to consider the ways that race and/or age might affect the experience of pregnancy, many participants acknowledged the social judgment that is levelled against pregnant Aboriginal women. As Christine put it, "society leads you to think ... a Native person who gets pregnant is a bad, bad thing. Don't do it. A white person that gets pregnant, it's okay... society can deal with it."

Social Differences and Experiences with Health Experts

As I spoke with women about their experiences with health experts during their pregnancies, women rarely questioned the importance of seeing a doctor regularly throughout their pregnancy. Indeed, many women felt "cared for" in proportion to the medical monitoring that they received. Across social differences, most women felt that regular visits to doctors during pregnancy were important to make sure that "everything was going okay" and, particularly, that the baby was okay.

While women felt that it was important to visit doctors throughout the pregnancy, most descriptions of typical visits to doctors suggested a certain passivity on the part of women in the sense that, while women may not have fully known the reasons for monitoring procedures or for doctors' decisions, they accepted medical authority over their bodies during pregnancy. The doctor-patient relationship emerged as one of unequal power in the sense that doctors had access to a culturally authoritative form of knowledge that women did not. As Christine commented:

> Because I'm not a doctor and I don't know what the ... you know what you're supposed to do, what you're not supposed to do [...] I had no idea what was going on, so I just went with what they said. If they told me to come in, I'd come in. If they told me to go for an ultrasound, I would go for an ultrasound. It's just what you do.

Yet, while the doctor-patient relationship emerged as one of unequal power in which women were compelled to acquiesce to medical authority because it is just "what you do," women did not always feel themselves to be without any sense of agency in these relationships. Rather, the degree of agency that women felt in the context of medical monitoring was affected by at least two important factors. The first of these factors was the quality of their relationship with their doctor.

The effect of the quality of women's relationships with health care professionals on women's sense of agency emerged in the data as women's visits to doctors during their pregnancies tended to fall into two categories of experience. For some women, visits to the doctor during pregnancy were positive experiences that provided reassurance and a sense that they were "cared for." In these cases, women felt the ability to ask questions and voice concerns. In other cases, visits to doctors were negative experiences during which women felt faceless and rushed through. In these cases, women felt like "a file" or a number and did not feel as though their concerns had been addressed. Whether women felt like a "file," or whether they felt cared for and listened to, did not appear to have any obvious relationship with social difference. Rather, whether women felt "cared for" or "like a file" appeared to depend on their ability to find and remain with a doctor that they felt comfortable with—which itself seemed to depend simply on whether or not women could find a caring general practitioner or whether or not they were referred to an obstetrician that they felt comfortable with.

The second important factor that could affect women's agency in doctor-patient relationships was social connectedness, which appeared to have the potential to enhance women's ability to reflexively utilize health experts or health expertise. This emerged in the data as instances where women received or shared information with each other that could enhance their own knowledge base about the expertise that doctors had to offer. For example, Kari, who took Diclectin (a drug that eases nausea) during her pregnancy, was able to share this information with her sister, who also experienced nausea. Kari was thus able to counsel her sister to ask her doctor for Diclectin. Similarly, when I spoke with Marie about her sources of information during her pregnancy, she revealed to me that she had learned through speaking with other moms at a community centre that Materna, a prenatal vitamin frequently recommended by doctors, was making many of the women there sick. Marie thus declined to take the vitamin when her doctor recommended it.

While social connectedness could affect women's knowledge base as they interacted with health care providers, factors such as youth and Aboriginal identity could affect the treatment women received from health workers. When I asked participants if age could affect the treatment women received from health care workers during their pregnancy, the answer was sometimes a tentative, and sometimes a definite, "yes." However, the specific contours of treatment differentials based on age did not clearly emerge. Thus, some women who were older when they were pregnant asserted that they had been treated with "more respect" than women they knew who were younger, while some younger women indeed felt that they themselves had been treated with less respect. Some women who were older suggested that younger women received "less attention." Still other women who were younger suggested that doctors "talked down" to them. While the contours of the negative treatment accorded young pregnant women emerged only vaguely, it appeared that this treatment was linked, at least in women's minds, to the lack of respect accorded young women more generally, and to the social judgment that surrounds teen pregnancy. It also appeared in this data set that the negative treatment accorded young pregnant women was a phenomenon that occurred when women were interacting with strangers and not with their regular doctors.

While women linked negative treatment based on age to the social judgment that surrounds teen pregnancy, in the experiences of some of the Aboriginal women I interviewed, Aboriginal identity could become a physical marker that suggested something "pathological" about a woman's behaviour or background. Thus, in an example of racism as intensified surveillance, Kari reported to me that she has never experienced any racism in the health care system, but that her friends tell her that she "looks white." However, she related a story of intensified surveillance when she took a friend to the hospital:

> ... but she looks Native and that's probably why they like grilled her, you know...trying to find out if she drank during her pregnancy. You know, I mean...I was surprised that they even...I mean they drilled her and like hard...

A process in which "race" becomes a physical marker of pathology was revealed in a particularly clear way in the experiences of two Aboriginal women who had non-Aboriginal mothers. Both of these women described experiencing discriminatory attitudes from health care workers; however, these discriminatory attitudes disappeared when they visited the hospital with their non-Aboriginal mothers. For example, when Sheila related her experiences of the negative societal judgment that is directed at young, pregnant Aboriginal women, I asked her if she ever felt that judgment in the health care system as well. In another example of racism as intensified surveillance, Sheila replied:

> In the health care system, yes. I do. Especially if some of those nurses are working their double shifts or if they're in some of their moods that they're in going there...it's "is this your third or fourth child"... you know, they expect that right away from you . . ."no this is my first!" But...do you do drugs...do you drink...do you smoke. I know some of these questions are what they're supposed to ask, but they direct it toward you like this is what you're doing. You know... and I'm just thinking...you're judging me and you don't know me... you know...they ask the questions with my second one "well...are

you still drinking, are you still smoking, are you doing drugs . . ." [. . .] But I noticed it was different when I would have my mother with me. My mother... she's Caucasian. I'm only half Aboriginal. And they wouldn't ask me those questions when I was there with my mom. They wouldn't...they would just ask me you know...what's the problem... and I see this is your first.

DISCUSSION

The results of this study indicate that as women interact with expert knowledge and health experts during their pregnancies, the extent of agency or regulation they experience is sometimes, but not always, affected by social differences such as age and Aboriginal identity. In this study, the potential for expert knowledge to enhance women's agency is revealed through results that suggest that expert advice solicited from a variety of sources gave women a sense of preparedness. Women also linked knowledge of nutritional recommendations and "risks," such as smoking and drinking, to control over their own and their baby's health. Women's desire for "expert" knowledge, as well as women's associations between "expert" knowledge and agency, appeared to have no relationship to social differences such as age, income, or Aboriginal/ non-Aboriginal identity. Similar results have been recorded in other studies. For example, in interview research with 26 low-income women in Ontario, Wendy Sword (2003) found that all the women she spoke with expressed a need and desire for prenatal services and knowledge surrounding self-care (nutrition, exercise, etc.). The results of this research, together with the findings of Sword's study, suggest that ethnicity, income, and age make no difference to women's desire to solicit "expert" knowledge during pregnancy and that across social differences the appropriation of expert knowledge can increase women's sense of agency and control.

Yet, while most of the women in my study linked the appropriation of expert knowledge to a sense of agency or control in relation to their own and their baby's health, the notion that women are responsible for their baby's health appeared to underlie instances of guilt, self-blame, and a process of mutual surveillance related to women's adherence to "expert knowledge." The tendency of expert knowledge surrounding pregnancy to enact a process of mutual surveillance is also suggested by the findings of research conducted by Laury Oaks (2000) in the Baltimore-Washington DC area. In interviews with health professionals and laywomen about their perceptions of cigarette smoking during pregnancy, Oaks found that an overwhelming number of non-smokers harshly judged pregnant smokers. Significantly, negative assessments of pregnant women who smoked were predicated on the idea that every woman should assume responsibility for the health of her baby-to-be. The results of the present research, as well as the results of Oaks' study, support the Foucauldian insight that the proliferation of expert knowledge can work to regulate women's agency by compelling individuals to conform to "normal" behaviours and by pathologizing those who do not.

The findings of this study also suggest that women's agency in relation to health experts is reduced by the culturally authoritative status of expert knowledge. Across social differences, all women solicited the attention of health experts and rarely questioned the importance of regular monitoring during pregnancy. Ellen Lazarus's (1994) research into women's pregnancy experiences in the United States has produced similar findings. In interviews with women from both lower-class and middle-class backgrounds, during the early and late 1980s respectively, Lazarus (1994, p. 26) found that all women, regardless of social class or ethnicity, accepted the medical view of birth "that any number of things could go wrong and that ultimately they had to rely on professional knowledge and technological expertise to ensure they had done everything possible to have a healthy baby."

Interestingly, Lazarus also concluded that lower-class women had a reduced sense of agency in the context of doctor-patient relations in comparison with middle-class women. In Lazarus's U.S.-based study, most of the lower-income women had less insurance than middle-class women and were thus less likely to see and develop a relationship with a regular doctor. The impersonalized care that lower-income women received at clinics led to a reduced sense of agency and control in the context of doctor-patient relations. In the present study, while social difference did not appear in an obvious way to bear on women's ability to find and remain with a doctor they felt comfortable with, it is significant that impersonalized care could also lead to a reduced sense of agency, in that women who felt "like a file" did not feel the agency to ask questions or voice concerns.

Another important result of this study was the positive effect of social connectedness on women's agency to reflexively utilize or resist expert advice. This appeared in the data when women's social relationships with each other allowed them to share experiences and opinions about expert knowledge. Women were then able to incorporate each other's experiences with expert knowledge into their own personal evaluation of this knowledge—as in the case of Marie, who disregarded her doctor's recommendation to take Materna. This result suggests that the social and economic inequalities that may create a situation of isolation for some women may also underlie differential levels of agency and reflexivity in relation to health experts.

Finally, some results suggest that both youth and Aboriginal identity can lead to regulation in the form of intensified surveillance or negative treatment. However, women's income levels did not appear to affect the treatment women received in the health care system. The absence of results related to income in this respect warrants some discussion. One possibility may be that "income level" as a socially produced (and socially constructed) category is less "visible" than age or Aboriginal identity and, therefore, less likely to become a basis for discrimination or intensified surveillance.[3] Another possibility may be that income level is somewhat "visible" but that health care workers are less likely to discriminate on the basis of income. Of course, it is also possible that discrimination on the basis of women's income levels is present in the health care system, but simply was not detected by this study due to either the size of the sample or the themes covered by the questions.

Notwithstanding the absence of results related to income, as I spoke with women about the ways that age can affect treatment from health care professionals, it appeared at times that the social judgment that accompanies teen pregnancy was also present in the medical system, leading to negative treatment. As I spoke with women about the ways that "race" can affect treatment from health care professionals, it appeared that "race" itself could become a physical marker that suggested something "pathological" about a woman's behaviour or background. This could lead to both negative judgment and intensified surveillance.

There has been little research that focuses specifically on how ethnicity or age can affect pregnant women's experiences with health care providers; however, in a study published by the British Columbia Centre of Excellence for Women's Health in 2000, Annette Brown, Jo-Anne Fiske, and Geraldine Thomas conducted qualitative interviews with women from a Carrier First Nation reserve community in British Columbia about their experiences with mainstream health care services. Among other negative experiences, such as feeling dismissed by health care providers or feeling negatively judged based on dress and speech style, participants also repeatedly shared experiences in which they felt that they were victims of discriminatory judgments levelled against Aboriginal women as mothers. The findings of Brown, Fiske, and Thomas suggest that the racism described by some Aboriginal women in my study may be illustrative of a broader phenomenon in the Canadian health care system. Indeed, it is significant that Brown, Fiske, and Thomas found that Aboriginal women encountered discrimination from health care workers based on negative judgments about their abilities as mothers, while some of the Aboriginal women in my study encountered discrimination from health care workers based on the assumption of "pathological" or "irresponsible" behaviour during pregnancy. Such findings suggest that social judgments related to who is "fit" or "unfit" to be pregnant are also connected to social judgments about who is "fit" or "unfit" to be a mother. In both cases, these judgments reappear in the health care system where Aboriginal women are assumed to be "irresponsible"—first, in relation to the health of their fetus and then, later on, in relation to the health of their child. In the British Columbia study, negative stereotypes and negative treatment could also lead to a reduced sense of trust in the health care system and a desire to avoid seeking health care altogether. While none of the women in my study reported that they avoided seeking health care through their pregnancies, this may constitute an area for further inquiry.

Indeed, the results of this research point to at least three questions that require further inquiry. A first direction for future research is suggested by results that indicate that the quality of women's relationships with their doctors can impact their agency to voice concerns and ask questions. While social differences, in the present study, did not appear to have an obvious effect on women's ability to form long-term and high-quality relationships with doctors, this does not preclude, but rather underlines, the importance of further research into the specific ways that social, economic, or geographic factors can enhance or impede women's ability to access high-quality, personalized medical care during their pregnancies. A second important direction for future research is suggested by results that indicated that the social surveillance of young women—and particularly young Aboriginal women—when they are pregnant can also manifest itself as negative treatment in the health care system. To the degree that the contours of this negative treatment did not always emerge clearly in women's experiences, future research ought to shift the focus to the attitudes and practices of health care workers themselves. Finally, while this research maintained a focus on the ways that social differences such as age, income, and Aboriginal identity can bear on women's encounters with expert knowledge, an important direction for future research is suggested by results that illustrate the importance of social connectedness to women's ability to respond to health experts with autonomy and reflexivity. These results point to the usefulness of research that expands the focus to include a more detailed exploration into the ways that the broader set of relationships and circumstances of women's lives can facilitate or inhibit agency and reflexivity as women interact with, appropriate, or resist expert knowledge and intervention during their pregnancies.

NOTES

1. Because one of the aims of this study was to explore how Aboriginal identity could impact women's experiences with expert knowledge and health "experts," women identified as "Aboriginal" were women who identified themselves as Aboriginal or identified with at least one Aboriginal group (that is, North American Indian, Inuit, Metis). Women identified as "non-Aboriginal" are women who did not identify in any of these ways.

2. "Poverty lines" are a set of low-income cut-offs defined by Statistics Canada "below which a household may be said to live in straitened circumstances" (Ross, Shillington, & Lockhead, 1994). As defined by Statistics Canada, the low-income cut-off for a given year and household size is a household income that corresponds to only 20 percent more than the amount of income necessary for food, clothing, and shelter (Ross, Shillington, & Lockhead, 1994). In the socio-demographic portion of the interview, I asked women to estimate their household income during their pregnancies within a $5,000 range (that is, $0–5,000, $5,001–10,000, $10,001–15,000, etc.). Taking the year and the household size into consideration, I classified women as living "near or below the poverty line" if their household income fell within or below the $5,000 range within which the poverty line was located.

3. It would be incorrect to imply that income is not always "physically visible." Pierre Bourdieu (1984), for example, has argued that social class (which is related to income) manifests itself in an individual's dress, speech style, tastes, and mannerisms. However, none of the participants in this study recalled or related stories in which they felt their income level was physically visible or in which they felt discriminated against on the basis of their social class.

REFERENCES

Arcury, T. A., & Quandt, S. A. (1999). Participant recruitment for qualitative research: A site-based approach to community research in complex societies. *Human Organization, 52*(2), 128–133.

Bourdieu, P. (1984). *Distinction: A social critique of the judgment of taste.* Cambridge, MA : Harvard University Press.

Armstrong, D. (1995). The rise of surveillance medicine. *Sociology of Health and Illness, 17*(3), 393–404.

Barker, K. K. (1998). A ship upon a stormy sea: The medicalization of pregnancy. *Social Science and Medicine, 47*(8), 1067–1076.

Beck, U. (1999). *World risk society.* Oxford: Blackwell.

Brown, A., & Smye, V. (2002). A post-colonial analysis of health care discourses addressing Aboriginal women. *Nurse Researcher, 9*(3), 28–41.

Brown, A. J., Fiske, J., & Thomas, G. (2000). First Nations women's encounters with mainstream health care services and systems. Vancouver: British Columbia Centre of Excellence for Women's Health.

Campbell, J. C. (2001). Abuse during pregnancy: A quintessential threat to maternal and child health: So when do we start to act? *Journal of the American Medical Association, 164*(11), 1578–1579.

Dyck, R., Klomp, H., Tan, L. K., Turnell, R. W., & Boctor, M. A. (2002). A comparison of rates, risk factors, and outcomes of gestational diabetes between Aboriginal and non-Aboriginal women in the Saskatoon Health District. *Diabetes Care, 25*(3), 487–492.

Feldman, P. J., Dunkel-Schetter, C., Sandman, C. A., & Wadhwa, P. D. (2000). Maternal social support predicts birth weight and fetal growth in human pregnancy. *Psychosomatic Medicine, 62*, 715–725.

Foucault, M. (1976). Governmentality. *m/f, 3*, 5–21.

Foucault, M. (1990). *The history of sexuality.* New York: Random House.

Foucault, M. (1995). *Discipline and punish.* New York: Random House.

Giddens, A. (1990). *The consequences of modernity.* Stanford, CA: Stanford University Press.

Giddens, A. (1999). Risk and responsibility. *Modern Law Review, 62*(1), 1–10.

Kramer, M. S., Seguin, L., Lydon, J., & Goulet, L. (2000). Socio-economic disparities in birth outcome: Why do the poor fare so poorly? *Paediatric and Perinatal Epidemiology, 14*, 194–210.

Lazarus, E. S. (1994). What do women want?: Issues of choice, control, and class in pregnancy and childbirth. *Medical Anthropology Quarterly, 8*(1), 25–46.

Lofland, J., & Lofland, L. H. (1995). *Analyzing social settings: A guide to qualitative observation and analysis.* Belmont, CA: Wadsworth.

Luo, Z.-C., Wilkins, R., Platt, R. W., & Kramer, M. S. (2004). Risks of adverse pregnancy outcomes among Inuit and North American Indian women in Quebec, 1985–97. *Paediatric and Perinatal Epidemiology, 18*, 40–50.

McDermott, R. (1998). Ethics, epidemiology, and the thrifty gene: Biological determinism as a health hazard. *Social Science and Medicine, 47*(9), 1189–1195.

Miles, M. B., & Huberman, M. A. (1994). *Qualitative data analysis.* Thousand Oaks, CA: Sage.

Mitchinson, W. (1998). Agency, diversity, and constraints: Women and their physicians, Canada, 1850–1950. In S. Sherwin (Ed.), *The politics of women's health: Exploring agency and autonomy* (pp. 122–149). Philadelphia: Temple University Press.

Mitchinson, W. (2002). *Giving birth in Canada, 1900–1950.* Toronto: University of Toronto Press.

Morgan, K. P. (1998). Contested bodies, contested knowledges: Women, health, and the politics of medicalization. In S. Sherwin (Ed.), *The politics of women's health: Exploring agency and autonomy* (pp. 83–121). Philadelphia: Temple University Press.

Muhajarine, N., & D'Arcy, C. (1999). Physical abuse during pregnancy: Prevalence and risk factors. *Canadian Medical Association Journal, 160*(7), 1007–1011.

Murphy, C. C., Schei, B., Myhr, T. L., & Du Mont, J. (2001). Abuse: A risk factor for low birth weight? A systemic review and meta-analysis. *Journal of the American Medical Association, 164*(11), 1567–1572.

Oakley, A. (1984). *The captured womb: A history of the medical care of pregnant women.* Oxford and New York: Blackwell.

Oaks, L. (2000). Smoke filled wombs and fragile fetuses: The social politics of fetal representation. *Signs, 26*(1), 63–108.

O'Neil, J., Reading, J. R., & Leader, A. (1998). Changing the relations of surveillance: The development of a discourse of resistance in Aboriginal epidemiology. *Human Organization, 57*(2), 230–237.

PHAC (Public Health Agency of Canada). (2008). *The sensible guide to a healthy pregnancy.* Accessed September 2008, from http://www.healthycanadians.gc.ca/hp-gs/guide_e.html

PHAC (Public Health Agency of Canada). (2000). *Pro-action, postponement, and preparation/ support: A framework for action to reduce the rate of teen pregnancy in Canada.* Paper prepared for the CAPC/CPNP National Projects Fund.

Peterson, A. R. (1996). Risk and the regulated self: The discourse of health promotion as politics of uncertainty. *Australian and New Zealand Journal of Sociology, 32*(1), 44–57.

Poudrier, J. (2007). The geneticization of Aboriginal diabetes and obesity: Adding another scene to the story of the thrifty gene. *Canadian Review of Sociology and Anthropology*, 44(2), 237–261.

Rose, N., & Miller, P. (1992). Political power beyond the State: Problematics of government. *British Journal of Sociology*, 43(2), 173–205.

Rose, N. (1993). Government, authority, and expertise in advanced liberalism. *Economy and Society*, 22(3), 283–299.

Ross, D. P., Shillington, E. R., & Lockhead, C. (1994). *The Canadian fact book on poverty 1994*. Ottawa: Canadian Council on Social Development.

Ruhl, L. (1999). Liberal governance and pre-natal care: Risk and regulation in pregnancy. *Economy and Society*, 28(1), 95–117.

Shim, J. K. (2000). Bio-power and racial, class, and gender formation in biomedical knowledge production. *Research in the Sociology of Health Care*, 17(1), 173–195.

Sword, W. (2003). Prenatal care use among women of low income: A matter of taking care of self. *Qualitative Health Research*, 13(3), 319–322.

Wenman, W. M., Joffres, M. R., & Tataryn, I. V. (2004). A prospective cohort study of pregnancy risk factors and birth outcomes in Aboriginal women. *Canadian Medical Association Journal*, 171(6), 585–589.

Williams, S. J., & Calnan, M. (1996). The "limits" of medicalization? Modern medicine and the lay populace in "late" modernity. *Social Science and Medicine*, 42(12), 1609–1620.

Zola, I. (1972). Medicine as an institution of social control. *Sociological Review*, 20(4), 487–504.

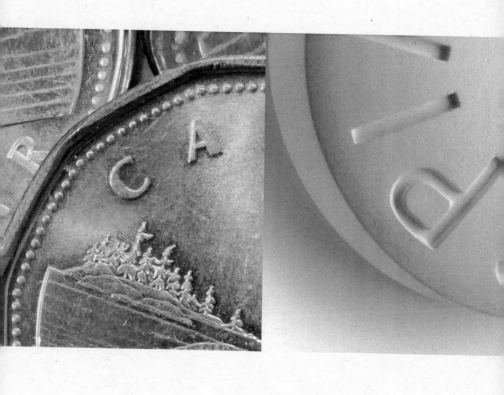

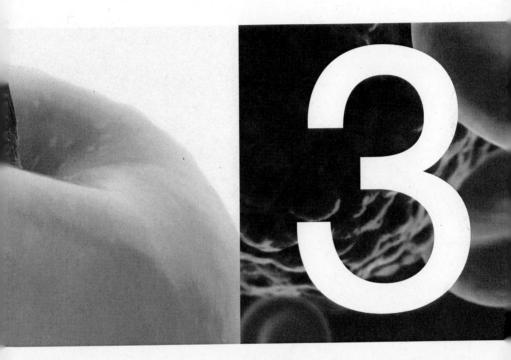

POPULATION HEALTH IN PRACTICE

Dragon Boat Racing as an Alternative Type of Support for Women Living with Breast Cancer

Rhona Shaw

Breast cancer remains the most common cancer among Canadian women.[1] One in nine women is expected to develop the disease during her lifetime, and one in twenty-eight women will die of this disease (Canadian Cancer Society, 2004). Treatment protocols depend on where one lives and which health care professionals oversee one's care (Gillham, 1994). Moreover, after treatment, supportive care varies and is regarded by many women as less than ideal (Helgeson, Cohen, & Schulz, 2000).

A growing number of women dealing with the experience of breast cancer are turning to the sport of dragon boat racing as a source of after-treatment leisure and for social and emotional support. The dragon boat racing phenomenon among women with breast cancer first began in Vancouver, BC, and was a research initiative of a Canadian sports medicine practitioner. The intention was to challenge the predominant medical opinion that women recovering from treatment for breast cancer should abstain from repetitive and strenuous physical activity. Popular at the time was the belief that intensive upper body physicality would lead to the development of lymphedema, a painful and persistent swelling of the hand, arm, and torso regions (Harris et al., 2001; Harris & Niesen-Vertommen, 2000). So popular was this activity among the women research participants that they decided to form a team and continue to paddle.

It was in 1996, in Vancouver, that the first known team of dragon boat racers consisting of women living with breast cancer was formed (Unruh &

Elvin, 2004). Soon thereafter, word about the sport spread throughout the breast cancer community and a social movement was born. Participation rates in the sport among women living with breast cancer continue to rise (Parry, 2008). At present, it is estimated that there are over 93 breast cancer survivor dragon boat racing teams worldwide, including Canada, the United States, Australia, China, England, Italy, Malaysia, New Zealand, Poland, Singapore, and South Africa (Parry, 2008).

There are now several studies that have looked at the experience of dragon boating among women living with breast cancer. Some of these studies have addressed the impact of this activity on women's lives. In these studies, the focus has been on understanding post-treatment needs of women living with breast cancer (Mitchell & Nielsen, 2002), women's psychological well-being (Unruh & Elvin, 2004), and the role played by dragon boat racing on breast cancer survivorship as a lifelong, dynamic process (Parry, 2007). Other studies that have addressed the experience of survivor dragon boat racing have done so through a physiological-rehabilitative lens. These include a study on exercise adherence within a theoretical model of exercise promotion (focusing on issues of non-compliance behaviours) (Courneya, Blanchard, & Laing, 2001), another regarding health-related quality of life with a focus on team cohesiveness (Culos-Reed, Shields, & Brawley, 2005), and three on the minimizing of risk and management of lymphedema (Harris & Niesen-Vertommen, 2000; Lane, Jespersen, & McKenzie, 2005; McKenzie, 1998). However, to date, there appear to be no studies that focus specifically on the social and emotional support functions and dynamics of this activity for women living with breast cancer.

As an important determinant of health, social support can have a positive effect on physical, psychological, emotional, and spiritual health and well-being (Broadhead et al., 1983; Glover & Parry, 2008; Schwarzer & Leppin, 1991). One important way in which social support can be provided is through participation in leisure and sporting activities. There is a growing body of literature demonstrating that regular participation in these endeavours as part of a social activity can help the facilitation of coping with life stressors, which can have innoculative and buffering effects (Coleman & Iso-Ahola, 1993; Coleman, 1993; Isho-Ahola & Park, 1996; Iwasaki & Mannell, 2000a, 2000b). According to Kleiber, Hutchinson and Williams (2002), "Leisure in its companionate and friendship forms, and through social activities, clearly has the potential to provide people with feelings of social support and a decreased sense of loneliness and isolation" (p. 222). However, little is known about the supportive role of leisure following a negative life experience like that of breast cancer, including the character and extent of leisure's usefulness in the coping process, which thus needs to be better understood (Hutchinson et al., 2003).

In this paper, I offer some preliminary findings on the nature and kinds of social and emotional support offered to women living with breast cancer who regularly participate in the physically intense sport of survivor dragon boat racing.

THEORETICAL FRAMEWORK

This paper is informed by a "critical interactionism," which is a theoretical perspective that emphasizes human agency and the interpretive processes through which meanings are constructed. It attends to the structural inequalities that mediate these processes, including gender inequalities. Critical interactionism blends symbolic interactionism and critical feminist theory.

As a perspective, symbolic interactionism focuses on the emergent, multiple, and complex ways in which people purposively create and make sense of their life-worlds in tandem with others (Prus, 1996). Although an important approach to an understanding of social life, social interactionism has been criticized by feminists for its indifference to the conditions of women's material and daily lives. Often ignored are the gendered practices and social relationships of power that constitute and shape women's life-worlds. While feminist scholarship shares with symbolic interactionism an interest in the lived experiences of social actors, particularly women, many feminists argue that what is needed is an approach that makes visible "the structures, practices, and inequities of gender social order" (Lorber, 2005, p. 11).

This paper marries these two perspectives so that the focus is on the gendered nature of social life, and how practical and everyday practices sustain or disrupt gender inequalities. I argue that in order to understand women's experiences of survivor dragon boat racing as an alternative form of social and emotional support for women living with breast cancer, two important contexts need to be considered. The first is that they are participating in this activity as women living with a life-threatening and often disabling disease, rather than as "well" women who are interested in dragon boating racing as a leisure activity per se. The second is that they are also women who live in a gender-stratified world where inequitable social relationships and cultural practices continue to shape their access to, participation in, and experiences of leisure and organized sport. Each of these contexts plays a critical role in shaping and mediating women's support experiences of this activity.

METHODS

The study was conducted between July 2002 and September 2007 among women who make up a breast cancer survivor dragon boat racing team located in a mid-sized urban centre in southwestern Ontario, Canada. Two data collection techniques were utilized in this study.

The first technique consisted of face-to-face, in-depth interviews that became more open-ended as they proceeded, as participants were encouraged to tell their own stories. Unscheduled prompts and follow-up questions were also utilized in order to elicit a breadth and depth in responses (Breakwell, 1995). This was to allow women to "reveal in their own words their view of their entire life, or part of it, or some aspect of themselves" (Bogdon & Taylor, 1975, p. 6). Of the 31 women interviewed, 26 tapes were transcribed—this owing to time and financial constraints—and used in this study. The interviews were transcribed verbatim and were read and reread in order to identify recurrent themes and sub-themes both within and between participants' accounts.

A second technique, participant observation, which is "characterised by a period of intense social interaction between the researcher and the subjects, in the milieu of the latter" (Bogdon & Taylor, 1975, p. 5), was also employed and continued for five years. The decision to include participant observation as a research technique was an important one because it allowed me intimate access to the group. This technique also helped to contextualize the themes that emerged in the women's interviews, it allowed me to connect with the women in ways that established trusting relationships, and it provided me with a much fuller understanding of their experiences of breast cancer and survivor dragon boat racing. As an "observer-participant," I took on an active membership role and became "more involved in the setting's central activities, assuming responsibilities that advance the group, but without fully committing [to] the members' values and goals" (Adler & Adler, 1994, p. 380). Regular contact and interaction with the group as a whole began in January 2003 when the team began their winter training for the racing season. These training sessions consisted of weekly weight workouts and paddling sessions at a local swimming pool. I also joined the team for the biweekly on-water paddling practices that began mid-May of that same year. I participated in these activities with the team regularly and also joined the small but regular group of women for drinks at a local pub after pool and paddling practices. In addition, I attended various team activities and travelled with the team to many of their regular season dragon boat competitions. Participant observation ended after the 2007 season.

THE GROUP

As a group, this team of dragon boat racers was fairly homogenous, including the group of 26 women whose interviews were used for this study. Of the 26 women interviewed, 22 were married and four were either single or never married. All but one of the women identified themselves as heterosexual, while one woman stated that she was neither heterosexual nor homosexual. At the time of the interviews, the women's ages ranged between 29 and 73 years. All of the women were of the Christian faith except one woman who said that she was agnostic. All of the interviewees but two identified as Canadian, and with further probing, identified themselves as either European or Anglo-Saxon. There were no women of colour involved with this group at the time of the interviews. Half of the women had attended or completed university, while nine had attended or completed college, and four had completed high school. The annual combined family incomes ranged between $20,000 CDN and $100,000+ CDN. The women of this particular group were white, well-educated, affluent, and professional—a demographic that appears to be characteristic of most breast cancer support and self-help groups (Gray et al., 1997), as well as women's athletic teams (Deem, 1987; Sternfeld, Ainsworth, & Quesenberry, 1999).

At the time of writing, three of the women interviewed have died as a result of their cancer metastasizing, and another four have been treated for localized recurrences. The average age of the women interviewed was 50, the average age at cancer diagnosis was 43, and the average time since diagnosis was seven years. In terms of breast cancer treatments, two women had bilateral mastectomies, four had lumpectomies, nine had segmental mastectomies, and ten had total mastectomies. Adjuvant treatments varied and depended on each woman's diagnosis. Seven women received radiation therapy, nine received chemotherapy, and six women received both. Nine women were taking Tamoxifen, a drug used to treat and manage women's breast cancer. Five of the women had reconstructive surgery. Several had a range of other conditions they were dealing with besides breast cancer, including fibromyalgia, lupus, scoliosis, arthritis, and lower back problems; some had been treated for other cancers such as ovarian, uterine, and thyroid. Five of the women interviewed were unable to paddle regularly because of health conditions; the remaining 21 were symptom-free throughout the time I was with them.

FINDINGS

Dragon boat racing is an intense physical activity that involves the development of upper body strength and cardiovascular stamina. Practices involve long hours of endurance training as well as sets of exercises that develop physical (upper body) power and speed.

The majority of those who joined the dragon boat team were women who had been physically active intermittently throughout most of their adult lives and who enjoyed physical activity for its own sake and not simply as a means of keeping body weight down and keeping slim. Many women had prior experience more specifically with water sports such as canoeing, kayaking, and water-skiing. Some described themselves as "water people." Part of the appeal of dragon boating for many of them had to do with the fact that it was a water-based leisure activity. However, the majority of women interviewed lacked team sport experience, and most had not participated in athletic pursuits that required physical training in order to compete.

For all of the women, however, dragon boating came to represent so much more than merely the opportunity to participate in an exciting and challenging sport. There were a number of recurrent and overlapping themes that pertained to support that emerged in the women's discussions of dragon boat racing. These included dragon boat racing as an alternative type of social support, support through friendship, and support through safe spaces.

AN ALTERNATIVE TO TRADITIONAL FORMS OF BREAST CANCER SUPPORT
By becoming regular members of the team, many of the women in the group interviewed came to count on their fellow team members for both social and emotional support and thought of the team as a support group.

"We call ourselves a floating support group." (Lola)

However, in several of the women's responses it was evident that not all regarded all support groups as "created equally," and for these women the dragon boat team offered them support of a different sort. Many of the women interviewed had been a part of conventional support groups for many years and benefited from their association with such groups, but found themselves wanting something different. Their participation in dragon boat racing did not necessarily represent a rejection of traditional forms of support, but rather that they were seeking out an alternative. Others, however, had difficulty with conventional groups from the start, finding them "heavy" and "depressing," and felt in need of something else. For example, Macaulay admitted that she was put off by what she saw as the "poor me" atmosphere that permeated the traditional peer support group she had once tried:

"I went to one of those (support groups). They were awful. A lot of the girls in the group went to another one and hated it. [*Did they say why?*] They were so down. I went to one and it was like "poor me." It was awful. Oh, and I'm like why are we here?.... Oh, the room was dark and everybody was sad and it was all horror stories. I'm thinking eww, yuck! How could you sit through it? Isn't this depressing? Why would you come back?"

Similarly, Mighty Mouse recounted her previous experience with a support group:

"We just come to it at a different angle than sitting in a group. [*And just talking?*] Yeah, well, just sitting and I went to some of the support groups for lupus and it really turned me off. You know as far as they are concerned you should be lying in your house just waiting to die type of deal and "Oh I can't do this and I can't do that . . ." And it was that, that made me stay away from regular breast cancer support groups too because I didn't want to sit and just hear the sad stories... And still dealing with it, but in a really positive, very upbeat sort of way."

The difference the women experienced in the dragon boat team as a source of support was in the activity-oriented premise and focus of the group. They saw the team as being about "doing" rather than "talking," and about getting on with life in spite of having breast cancer. They also emphasized the fun they had as a team, as well as the hard work they put into their training and the laughs they shared with one another.

"It's just a wonderful group of women who love to laugh." (Lola)

Some women were impatient with those who preferred to see themselves as victims or who exhibited a "why me God?" attitude. Talking about one's breast cancer experiences in a woeful or self-pitying manner was not tolerated, nor was it indulged. The attitude among some was "You've got five minutes to get over it" (Bette). The ethos of the group is to "get on with it," to stay focused on the positive, and to live life to the fullest because one is never sure how much time one has left.

"People will often say: 'Why me?' I never did. Why not me? Why should I be any different from anybody else? Why should I be special?" (Babs)

"There's also a whole group of people who need to be pulled up by just what this dragon boat does, and to be there for each other. We're not talking breast cancer; lots of times it's never mentioned in a night, in any night. But you also know that there's somebody there to give you a hug if the hug is needed or to say to you, hey." (Gabby)

This is not to say that the women were not compassionate, nor understanding; they were. In fact, it is ironic given the pains that some of the women took to distinguish the team from conventional peer support groups that, in important ways, the team serves precisely the same functions as other types of support groups, including information exchange and emotional support. Regarding themselves as a "competitive breast cancer team on the water, but a support group on land," the support group/self-help role comes into play whenever someone requests information about treatment protocols or procedures, is diagnosed with recurrence of her cancer, or is facing death. Support takes many forms and ranges from cards and emails of encouragement to nursing care (several women on the team are nurses), to running errands, minding children, cleaning houses, and preparing meals.

Information exchange is done informally, with requests for information usually made via email or through announcements at the beginning of practices. Often women will approach each other or the team's founder, who happens to be a nurse and is married to a sports medicine doctor, before going to see their own doctors. Several women spoke of the difficulties they had talking candidly and openly to their doctors about their illness and treatment experiences. Thus, the team provides its members with information, resources, care, and alternative approaches and perspectives concerning their illness experience that they feel they cannot get from their own cancer care practitioners.

"No, no, you don't get much from doctors." (Lady Di)

"They (the doctors) don't know how to deal with it. So it's the first place we go (the team) when we've got questions before we make that final decision to go to the doctor. A lot of time, they'll come and say 'I've got this what do you think?' And we'll say, whatever. And that way we're not going out there and they're labelling us as nuts. [*Or as hypochondriacs.*] Yeah, because that's not fun either. And it gives us a little more self worth." (Mighty Mouse)

Mighty Mouse's comment speaks to the uneasy relationships that many women have with their doctors and the need this creates to have their concerns legitimated. The dragon boat team functions in many ways to meet women's needs in this area.

However, it is important to emphasize that the support function of the group expresses itself in the context of the physical *raison d'être* of the team and that the dragon boat racing, in fact, becomes the means through which support—when it is needed—is delivered. In the following statements, Martha and Esther expressed it well:

> "I like the physical aspect of it rather than if it had been just a social group with people who were dragon boaters. But the fact that I could go every week and work on the exercise and I didn't even have to talk to anyone or I didn't have to be part of this, like, I ended up being part of the team and I'm very happy to be part of the team. But I wasn't, like, I wasn't interested in the touchy feely and I would have run the other way." (Martha)

> "It sounded exciting to me physically...I could see all these other pluses and now it's such a turn-on, of course the paddling is still a turn-on, I love that, but you go there and you talk to people and you find out if somebody is having a bad day or a good day. You get involved in their lives. The caring starts as you get to know people and then it really becomes so much more." (Esther)

The dragon boat team as a physically oriented support/self-help organization offers women positive alternatives and choices. They can participate in the group and receive emotional support from others that helps them adapt to life with breast cancer, or they can participate in the group for the physical activity and for the physical and health benefits that the strenuous exercise provides.

SUPPORT THROUGH FRIENDSHIP

The team aspect of the women's involvement in dragon boat racing also contributes to the strong bonds of friendship that develop and provides women with an important source of emotional and social support. Team sport has the capacity to facilitate female bonding, friendship, and a sense of sisterhood through the sharing of a similar interest in physical activity and through goal-orientated competition that emphasizes support and co-operation (Blinde, Taub, & Han, 1994; Theberge, 1987; Young, 1997). It is not surprising, under these circumstances, to find that the women bonded and pursued deep and meaningful friendships with each other:

> "The friendship bond gets better and deeper with every year and with every changing health situation that involves giving of oneself emotionally to one another." (Esther)

"Oh I just have a good time. I just enjoy it. It's like an extended family. Again it's a thing that I don't have, sisters. It's just, I love it!" (Meryl)

In describing their friendships the women stressed the base of understanding and shared experiences that make these relationships so powerful. Bette pointed out that this base, at least in terms of their breast cancer, is there whether it is openly talked about or not:

"It's nice to be among women who've had breast cancer so you're all coming from the same spot, but they don't talk about breast cancer. It's like friends you went to university with. You all knew you were from the same university with the same experience.... And I know that if I ever needed to talk about anything, that there are women that I could go to, that I could discuss it with. And it's a nice feeling."

When in the company of each other, the women felt that they did not have to maintain any pretence, either in terms of what they said or in terms of how they looked. For many, there was a reluctance to talk to "outsiders," even if they were significant and caring others, for fear of alarming them or of not being understood. There was also reluctance, in relation to the outside world, to reveal the scars of their surgeries or other side effects of their treatments. Among themselves, however, the women felt they could be "who they are":

"What keeps me coming back is the friendships, the workout, the people who don't care how I look. Just that I am there week after week to share a smile, a hug and a story with someone who can relate to whatever I am going through." (Charlie)

"You can talk to them about anything because they've been through it, they've been through the major thing like you have. You go on and whine but you know that if you really need to speak to someone there's always somebody there." (Lola)

SUPPORT THROUGH SAFE SPACES

Another critical support function that the dragon boat team serves has to do with the "safe space" it provides for team members, in both a literal and figurative sense. The previous section on friendship touched on the possibilities that the strong bonds between the women create for them an opportunity to "be themselves," and to share their experiences, hopes, dreams, fears, and terrors with each other with the expectation that they will be understood.

According to McKenzie and Crouch (2004), "cancer survivors' most profound feelings lie outside the acceptable limits of practical consciousness and will largely be debarred from expression in ordinary social intercourse which is constrained by routines of the natural attitude" (p. 143). Women are only too aware that talking about their breast cancer can disrupt and problematize social interaction. They also contend with others' lack of knowledge and understanding of what it is like to live with a life-threatening disease, and how life does not return to what it was after diagnosis and treatment (McKenzie & Crouch, 2004). Esmeralda put it like this:

> "So it was really weird how people looked at you, you know? They felt sorry for me. You just sort of have that label whether you like to admit it or not, you're labelled. [*And people don't know what to do or say to you.*] Yeah and that's what so comfortable about (the team) they take the stigma away and you can laugh and joke about your families. There's a bond I never thought I would have."

Suzanna, who at the time of her interview was dying, talked about how difficult it was for her to express herself to her family. She explained that they would not allow her to discuss her imminent death or to share with them her feelings about dying. The fact that she understood why this might be the case and that she did not doubt their love for her, however, did not make the situation easier for her to bear.

> "My family... expects me to be the same as I was. They don't give me a lot of leeway which is sometimes hurtful, but mostly, but at least they love me." (Suzanna)

Another dimension in which the team offers the women emotional and social support via a safe space is in terms of self-esteem and body image, which much of the popular and medical discourse about the loss of the female breast emphasizes as damaging consequences of this experience (Anderson, Woods, & Cyranowski, 1994; Bredin, 1999; Himes, 1994; Kraus, 1999; Wilmoth, 2001). The societal view of this experience puts women who have lost a breast to cancer in a position where it is expected, even demanded, that they feel anxiety about the loss and, further, that they exhibit this anxiety either by wearing a prosthesis or by undergoing breast reconstructive surgery. In other words, women are expected to take the necessary measures to represent to others a normalized feminine body that masks the telltale signs of their breast cancer and their breast loss (Lorde, 1980; Yadlon, 1997; Young, 1990).

These expectations and the consequences of transgressing them are part of women's breast cancer experiences. Macaulay recalled how female patrons at the fitness club where the team used to work out responded to the sight of the "breastlessness" of some of the team members. Several of the patrons were so disturbed by the sight of team members' disfigured bodies that they went to the club's management and complained about the team members changing their clothes in front of them.

> "Like we used to go to [name of the club] racquetball club but some of the ladies were upset that we got undressed in the locker room, we upset them. [*And they communicated that to you?*] They said that to the manager and we're no longer there. The disfigurement, it upset them, that we were disfigured and we were disrobing in front of them." (Macaulay)

When they are exclusively in each other's company, however, the women experience the freedom to "be who they are" in how they look, as well as in how they express themselves. They can be women living with breast cancer, women whose bodies are now marked or scarred. In this space, breast prostheses and other devices used to deny their breast cancer and normalize their bodies are not necessary. Many of the women experienced this as a burden from which they had been liberated. Gabby talked about the struggle over being able to express herself as a woman who was now single-breasted, and how her husband used to admonish her whenever she went without her prosthesis in public. However, when in the presence of the team she did not feel this normative pressure to hide her "lack" and instead felt the freedom to be herself as a women with one breast.

> "So now the only place I go without it [her prosthesis] is the dragon boat because I tried to. First of all I had to express myself, myself was nothing there [her missing breast], but then Clint [her husband] would say to me 'Gabby.' That's all he does. That means there's nothing there." (Gabby)

Similarly, Lucille drew attention to the team as a refuge.

> "The supportive people on the team and the feeling of sanctuary." (Lucille)

When in the company of each other, the women did not have to worry about embarrassing or offending others with their difference—as bald, disfigured—or with the fact that they had breast cancer. In these safe and protected spaces, the women are not only sheltered from, but can also challenge and resist, the critical gazes and comments of others. This aspect of their participation in the team is reflected clearly in an insightful comment made by Mimi. Mimi described the team as providing the women with a "power base," a position of both authority and solidarity among a group of women who all share a similar lived understanding—what it means to have breast cancer and what it is like to lose a breast (or breasts):

> "All of this might have been a totally, or would have been a totally different experience without the dragon boat because it has given you a power base to work from. If you were going through all of this as an isolated individual it would have been totally different. But being a part of this group where the joke is you can't wear your prosthesis on the boat because it weighs too much, it has to go overboard, it's a totally liberating thing. It allows you to be who you are, not who you're expected to be and that has been a huge bonus." (Mimi)

CONCLUDING COMMENTS

Reflecting on the women's support experiences as part of the dragon boat racing team, it is impossible to ignore the centrality of the two overlapping threads that provide the context for these experiences and which profoundly shape them—their breast cancer and the gendered contexts within which women live their lives.

First and foremost, these were women who were led to dragon boating as a result of a diagnosis of breast cancer. They were not women who had simply found an engaging and challenging leisure activity to participate in, or even women participating in dragon boat racing after treatment for a disease. They were women who came to dragon boat racing as individuals who had been diagnosed with, treated for, and were now living with, breast cancer. A diagnosis of breast cancer is the kind of experience that brings into stark relief the reality of one's mortality and the very real possibility of a premature death. Although not every woman diagnosed with breast cancer dies of the disease, one in three does. This means that even for those who ultimately survive, there is always the spectre of recurrence and death with all of the existential issues that these possibilities raise (Colyer, 1996; Payne, Sullivan, & Massie, 1996). A diagnosis of breast cancer can disrupt assumptions about one's daily life, including future expectations; for many, it initiates changes to one's sense of self (Arman & Rehnsfeldt, 2003).

Treatments for the disease can also assault and problematize physiological and biological processes, both during and long after treatments have ended (Love, 2000; Thomas-MacLean, 2004). Most women who are diagnosed with breast cancer receive a range of treatments (Reigle, 2006), which involve more than the amputation (in part or in whole) of the breast and surrounding breast tissue. Local and systemic treatments for breast cancer can be intensive, invasive, and toxic, depending on the number and types of treatments used. Treatments for breast cancer can give rise to a series of iatrogenic, chronic, and deleterious side effects (for example, fatigue, lymphedema, limited mobility, pain, hot flashes, compromised respiratory function, etc.) and can have implications for women's embodiment in both the short and longer term (Mustin, Katula, & Gill, 2002; Thomas-MacLean, 2005). Memories of these difficult and sometimes traumatic experiences of treatment linger and remain salient.

It is against this backdrop that the women experienced their participation on the dragon boat racing team as supportive, positive, and life-affirming. Along with the often unconditional support that they received from their teammates, the women also felt vital, alive, strong, and empowered. They could scarcely believe what they were accomplishing both individually and as a team. In how their bodies looked and in what those bodies could do, they found a reason to be proud. They could display those bodies among themselves without worrying about offending or upsetting others.

Also critical to an understanding of the participants' support experiences is women's location within broader gendered social relations and practices, including women's experiences of sport. In a variety of ways the women were dealing with expectations about their appearance, their availability to perform their traditional roles in relation to their families and others around them, and, particularly, their physical capabilities or lack thereof. Women's circumscribed roles often lead to a lack of a sense of entitlement to leisure and to taking time out for themselves—and away from their families—to pursue their own interests. There is a "feminine ethic of care," which women often internalize, that holds that, as women, they should nurture and seek to meet the needs of others at the expense of their own needs (Harrington, Dawson, & Bolla, 1992). For many women and girls, access to and participation in sport—especially activities that involve intense physicality—is limited (Fasting, 1987; Sleep & Wormald, 2001). An indifference to sport begins early in the lives of many young girls, and organized sport does not become an important part of the culture of girls and women in the same way it does for boys and men (Fasting, 1987; Sleep & Wormald, 2001). Medical and scientific discourses that typify women's bodies as incapable of withstanding the rigours of intense physicality and strenuous sport further limit women's access to and participation in sport (Hall, 2002).

From the experiences of this particular group of women, it is clear that leisure and sport-based activities can provide those who participate regularly with emotional and social support, which can aid in coping with stressors that are associated with living with a life-threatening disease. However, it is important to be clear that, although these women are participating in survivor dragon boat racing because of an interest in physical activity and of returning to and maintaining health, the support function of this leisure activity, even if it only emerges at critical moments, is a key identifying and organizing component of the team's intent and dynamic. Thus, the nature and kinds of relationships, including the forms of social and emotional support that can emerge, are based on a shared experience and understanding of what it is like to live with a life-threatening disease and may differ from the experiences of those who participate in non-illness themed leisure.

This paper offers preliminary findings on the nature and forms of social and emotional support that participation in breast cancer survivor dragon boat racing offers to those women who participate regularly. However, there is a need for further research into the self-help and support group function of this activity in terms of how support and care emerge, who becomes involved in organizing and carrying out this care, and how this care and support is regarded and experienced by family members. There is also a need to look at and compare the experiences of several breast cancer survivor teams in order to discern the similarities and differences between the groups and how care and support is organized and carried out across a ranges of experiences. Attention also needs to be paid to the similarities and differences that emerge between teams that are recreational and those that have become competitive and whether the move towards competitiveness impacts or problematizes the support function of this activity.

Finally, there are also interesting comparisons to be made and explored in terms of the self-help and support group function of other illness-themed physical activities, including the mediating role gender might play in the nature and types of supportive care that emerge.

NOTES

1. With the exception of non-melanoma skin cancer.

REFERENCES

Adler, P. A., & Adler, P. (1994). Observational techniques. In N. Denzin & Y. Lincoln (Eds.), *Handbook of qualitative research* (pp. 377–392). Thousand Oaks, CA: Sage Publications.

Anderson, B., Woods, X., & Cyranowski, J. (1994). Sexual self-schema as a possible predictor of sexual problems following cancer treatment. *The Canadian Journal of Human Sexuality, 3*(2), 165–170.

Arman, M., & Rehnsfeldt, A. (2003). The hidden suffering among breast cancer patients: A qualitative metasynthesis. *Qualitative Health Research, 13*(4), 510–527.

Blinde, E., Taub, D., & Han, L. (1994). Sport as a site for women's group and societal empowerment: Perspective from the college athlete. *Sociology of Sport Journal, 11*, 51–59.

Bogdon, R., & Taylor, S. (1975). *Introduction to qualitative research methods: A phenomenological approach to the social sciences.* Toronto: John Wiley and Sons.

Breakwell, G. (1995). Interviewing methods. In G. M. Breakwell, S. Hammond, & C. Fife-Shaw (Eds.), *Research methods in psychology* (pp. 232–253). London: Sage Publications.

Bredin, M. (1999). Mastectomy, body image and therapeutic massage: a qualitative study of women's experiences. *Journal of Advanced Nursing, 29*(5), 1113–1120.

Broadhead, E., Kaplan, B., James, S., Wagner, E., Schoenbach, V., Grimson, R., Heyden, S., Tibblin, G., & Gehlbach, S. (1983). The epidemiologic evidence for a relationship between social support and health. *American Journal of Epidemiology, 117*(5), 521–537.

Canadian Cancer Society. Breast Cancer Stats 2004. Accessed April 7, 2005, from http://www.cancer.ca/ccs/internet/standard/0,3182,3172_14435__langId-en,00.html

Coleman, D., & Iso-Ahola, S. (1993). Leisure and health: The role of social support and self-determination. *Journal of Leisure Research, 25*(2), 111–128.

Coleman, D. (1993). Leisure based social support, leisure dispositions and health. *Journal of Leisure Research, 25*(4), 350–361.

Colyer, H. (1996). Women's experience of living with cancer. *Journal of Advanced Nursing, 23*, 496–501.

Courneya, K., Blanchard, C., & Laing, D. (2001). Exercise adherence in breast cancer survivors training for a dragon boat race competition: A preliminary investigation. *Psycho-Oncology, 10*, 444–452.

Culos-Reed, N., Shields, C., & Brawley, L. (2005). Breast cancer survivors involved in vigorous team physical activity: Psychosocial correlates of maintenance participation. *Psycho-Oncology, 14*, 594–605.

Deem, R. (1987). Unleisured lives: Sport, in the context of women's leisure. *Women's Studies International Forum, 10*(4), 423–432.

Fasting, K. (1987). Sports and women's culture. *Women's Studies International, 10*(4), 361–368.

Gillham, L. (1994). Lymphoedema and physiotherapists: Control not cure. *Physiotherapy, 80*(12), 835–843.

Glover, T., & Parry, D. (2008). Friendships developed subsequent to a stressful life event: The interplay of leisure, social capital, and health. *Journal of Leisure Research, 40*(2), 208–230.

Gray, R., Fitch, M., Davis, C., & Phillips, C. (1997). A qualitative study of breast cancer self-help groups. *Psycho-Oncology, 6*(4), 279–289.

Hall, M. A. (2002). *The girl and the game. A history of women's sport in Canada.* Peterborough: Broadview Press.

Harrington, M., Dawson, D., & Bolla, P. (1992). Objective and subjective constraints on women's enjoyment of leisure. *Society and Leisure, 15*(1), 203–221.

Harris, S., & Niesen-Vertommen, S. (2000). Challenging the myth of exercise-induced lymphedema following breast cancer: A series of case reports. *Journal of Surgical Oncology, 74*, 95–99.

Harris, S., Hugi, M., Olivotto, I., & Levine, M. (2001). Clinical practice guidelines for the care and treatment of breast cancer: 11. Lymphedema. *Canadian Medical Association Journal, 164*(2), 191–197.

Helgeson, V., Cohen, S., & Schulz, R. (2000). Group support interventions for women with breast cancer: Who benefits from what? *Health Psychology, 19*(2), 107–114.

Himes, M. (1994). Cancer and sexuality: Shared personal stories. *The Canadian Journal of Human Sexuality, 3*(2), 95–106.

Hutchinson, S., Loy, D., Kleiber, D., & Dattilo, J. (2003). Leisure as a coping resource: Variations in coping with traumatic injury and illness. *Leisure Sciences, 25*, 143–161.

Isho-Ahola, S., & Park, C. (1996). Leisure-related social support and self-determination as buffers of stress-illness relationship. *Journal of Leisure Research, 28*(3), 169–187.

Iwasaki, Y., & Mannell, R. (2000a). Hierarchical dimensions of leisure stress coping. *Leisure Sciences, 22*, 163–181.

Iwasaki, Y., & Mannell, R. (2000b). The effects of leisure beliefs and coping strategies on stress-health relationship: A field study. *Leisure/Loisir, 24*(1–2), 3–57.

Kleiber, D., Hutchinson, S., & Williams, R. (2002). Leisure as a resource in transcending negative life events: Self-protection, self-restoration, and personal transformation. *Leisure Sciences, 24*, 219–235.

Kraus, P. (1999). Body image, decision making, and breast cancer treatment. *Cancer Nursing, 22*(6), 421–427.

Lane, K., Jespersen, D., & McKenzie, D. (2005). The effect of a whole body exercise programme and dragon boat training on arm volume and arm circumference in women treated for breast cancer. *European Journal of Cancer Care, 14*(4), 353–358.

Lorber, J. (2005). *Gender inequality: Feminist theories and politics.* (3rd ed.). Los Angeles: Roxbury Publishing.

Lorde, A. (1980). *The cancer journals.* San Francisco: Aunt Lute Books.

Love, S. (2000). *Dr. Susan Love's breast book.* (2nd ed.). Reading, MA: Perseus Books.

McKenzie, D. (1998). Abreast in a boat—a race against breast cancer. *Canadian Medical Association Journal, 159*, 376–378.

McKenzie, H., & Crouch, M. (2004). Discordant feelings in the lifeworld of cancer survivors. *Health: An Interdisciplinary Journal for the Social Study of Health, Illness and Medicine, 18*(2), 139–157.

Mitchell, T., & Nielsen, T. (2002). Living life to the limits. Dragon boaters and breast cancer. *Canadian Woman Studies, 21*(3), 50–58.

Mustin, K., Katula, J., & Gill, D. (2002). Exercise: Complementary therapy for breast cancer rehabilitation. *Women & Therapy, 25*(2), 105–118.

Parry, D. (2007). "There is life after breast cancer": Nine vignettes exploring dragon boat racing for breast cancer survivors. *Leisure Sciences, 29*(1), 53–69.

Parry, D. (2008). The contribution of dragon boat racing to women's health and breast cancer survivorship. *Qualitative Health Research, 18*(2), 222–233.

Payne, D., Sullivan, M., & Massie, M. (1996). Women's psychological reactions to breast cancer. *Seminars in Oncology, 23*(1), 89–97.

Prus, R. (1996). *Symbolic interaction and ethnographic research. Intersubjectivity and the study of lived human experience.* New York: SUNY Press.

Reigle, B. (2006). The prevention of disablement: A framework for the breast cancer trajectory. *Rehabilitation Nursing, 31*(4), 174–179.

Schwarzer, R., & Leppin, A. (1991). Social support and health: A theoretical and empirical overview. *Journal of Social and Personal Relationships, 8,* 99–127.

Sleep, M., & Wormald, H. (2001). Perceptions of physical activity among young women aged 16 and 17 years. *European Journal of Physical Education, 6,* 26–37.

Sternfeld, B., Ainsworth, B., & Quesenberry Jr., C. (1999). Physical activity patterns in a diverse population of women. *Preventive Medicine, 28,* 313–323.

Theberge, N. (1987). Sport and women's empowerment. *Women's Studies International Forum, 10*(4), 387–393.

Thomas-MacLean, R. (2004). Memories of treatment: The immediacy of breast cancer. *Qualitative Health Research, 14*(5), 628–643.

Thomas-MacLean, R. (2005). Beyond dichotomies of health and illness: Life after breast cancer. *Nursing Inquiry, 12*(3), 200–209.

Unruh, A., & Elvin, N. (2004). In the eye of the dragon: Women's experience of breast cancer and the occupation of dragon boat racing. *The Canadian Journal of Occupational Therapy, 71*(3), 138–149.

Wilmoth, M. (2001). The aftermath of breast cancer: An altered sexual self. *Cancer Nursing, 24*(4), 278–286.

Yadlon, S. (1997). Skinny women and good mothers: The rhetoric of risk, control, and culpability in the production of knowledge about breast cancer. *Feminist Studies, 23*(3), 645–677.

Young, I. M. (1990). Breasted experience. The look and the feeling. In *Throwing like a girl and other essays in feminist philosophy and social theory* (pp. 189–209). Indianapolis: Indiana University Press.

Young, K. (1997). Women, sport and physicality. *International Review for the Sociology of Sport, 32*(3), 297–305.

Integrating Population Health Promotion and Prevention: A Model Approach to Research and Action for Vulnerable Pregnant Women

Angela Bowen and Nazeem Muhajarine

Depression exacts a huge emotional and physical burden on women and their growing families. Unborn and newborn children are especially susceptible to the influence of their mothers' mental health and can experience lifelong problems as a result of unrecognized and untreated depression. Prenatal care usually follows a traditional biomedical model that focuses only on the physical well-being of the mother and her unborn baby. However, women's lives are complex and their problems are not necessarily only physical; many more factors can impact the health of the developing fetus. These other factors are not normally assessed by a traditional biomedical model.

For example, Jolene, a single mother of two young children living in an inner-city neighbourhood, finds herself unexpectedly pregnant. She experiences high levels of stress and a lack of social support. These less-than-optimal conditions may trigger symptoms of anxiety and depression, putting her and her unborn baby at risk for poor health outcomes at birth and beyond. A conventional biomedical approach may recognize, treat, and manage Jolene's anxiety and depression. However, in the past, in our community, there has been little attention paid to depression in pregnancy. An alternative integrated model of care grounded in population health and levels of prevention would not only identify and manage Jolene's physical health during pregnancy, with due care for the developing fetus, but also extend this care and advocacy as necessary for the life context in which Jolene finds herself.

This paper describes a model approach for research and action for pregnant women. It begins with background information about depression in pregnancy. We describe the "Feelings in Pregnancy and Motherhood Study," a study of depression in pregnant women living in socially high-risk conditions, conducted through the University of Saskatchewan. This paper also outlines an approach for working with health care providers and women themselves to enact changes in consultation and treatment practices to help women. The model incorporates two theoretical perspectives: first, the levels of prevention, which underlie the foundational rationale and implications of the study; and second, the population health perspective, which provides a framework for research questions, data collection, and interpretation of findings, as well as subsequent program and policy development.

BACKGROUND

Depression is an increasingly urgent public, mental, and population health problem (WHO, 2006). It is commonly defined as a negative emotional state during which an individual feels sad, lonely, or miserable, with a "lack of interest" in usual pleasurable activities (Blazer, 1999). According to the American Psychiatric Association, depression may be diagnosed if an individual displays five or more of the following symptoms in a two-week period: depressed mood most of the day; anhedonia (severely diminished interest or pleasure in activities); weight changes secondary to appetite changes; insomnia or hypersomnia; psychomotor changes (restless, agitated, or slowed); fatigue or diminished energy level; feelings of worthlessness or excessive or inappropriate guilt; decreased concentration and increased indecisiveness; and/or recurrent thoughts of death or suicide (American Psychiatric Association, 2000).

In 2000, the World Health Organization (WHO) ranked depression as the fourth greatest contributor to disability worldwide, responsible for 3.7 percent of the total global disease burden as determined by the Disability Adjusted Life Years (DALYs—sum of years of potential life lost due to premature mortality and the years of productive life lost due to disability) in both sexes in the 15–44 age group (Mathers et al., 2002; see also Cole et al., 2000). However, depression, according to the World Health Organization, is already the number one cause of disability in women worldwide (WHO, 2006).

One in five women seeking prenatal care in a primary care setting may experience depression in pregnancy, or soon after birth of the baby (Marcus et al., 2003). We have reported a prevalence of depression in pregnancy at 29.5 percent in women living in socially high-risk conditions (that is, low income and education, non-partnered, frequent transience from home to home) (Bowen & Muhajarine, 2006; Bowen et al., 2009). This is greater than the prevalence of other common physical prenatal problems that receive much medical attention, such as gestational diabetes (Spirito et al., 1992). Depression during pregnancy is of particular significance not just because of the consequences to the health of the mother, but also because of the potential deleterious effects on the developing fetus (Glover & O'Connor, 2002).

Barker, in his theory of the "foetal origins of adult disease," hypothesized that the prenatal environment exerts influences on fetal health that, in turn, impact the health of the adult many decades later (Barker, 1995). Therefore, increased understanding of the health determinants associated with depression in pregnancy is essential to reduce the intergenerational spread of the sequelae of depression, from mother to child and so forth.

The multiple effects of depression on the childbearing family are increasingly reported in the literature. Pregnant women who are depressed experience deteriorating social function, emotional withdrawal, and excessive concern about the pregnancy, and they worry more about their ability to parent (Murray, Cooper, & Hipwell, 2003; Norbeck & Tilden, 1983). The emotional withdrawal and disengagement from normal functions sometimes leads to further breakdown of the primary relationships women have formed, further threatening their social supports (Seto et al., 2005). Women who are depressed are more likely to use alcohol, drugs, and tobacco, and are less likely to have adequate prenatal care. All of these factors contribute to poor outcomes for the fetus, the baby, and the mother herself (Zuckerman et al., 1989; Bonari et al., 2004; Kahn, Certain, & Whitaker, 2002). Their pregnancies are more likely to end prematurely and have more obstetrical complications (Chung et al., 2001).

Infants whose mothers were depressed during pregnancy are at increased risk for preterm delivery, lower Apgar scores, lower birth weight, less frequency and shorter duration of breastfeeding, poorer weight gain, and increased admission to neonatal intensive care (Chung et al., 2001; Hellin & Waller, 1992; Murray & Cooper, 2003; Zuckerman et al., 1990). They score lower on development scales and have increased stress behaviours, less imitative behaviour, less mature sleep patterns, and more irritability (Field, 1997). Field believes this combination of factors indicates dysregulation in the infant and is likely to have a negative effect on mother-baby interaction and forming attachment (Field, 1997). As they grow, the children of mothers who are depressed experience more growth, psychological, behavioural, and developmental problems (for example, autism and criminality) than children of mothers who are not depressed (Caplan et al., 1989; Maki et al., 2003; Murray & Cooper, 2003; O'Connor et al., 2002; Wilkerson et al., 2002).

Women who are depressed in pregnancy are at increased risk for further and more severe depressive episodes, including postpartum depression, psychosis, and suicide (Blazer, 1999; Heron et al., 2004). Partners of women with postpartum depression are up to 50 percent more likely to be depressed themselves, especially if the woman is severely depressed (Goodman, 2004). There is no reason to expect that the same issue would not occur during pregnancy (Goodman, 2004).

The evidence about the consequences of depression in pregnancy on the developing fetus and growing child is compelling. Effective treatments for depression are available, including interpersonal therapy, support groups, electroconvulsive therapy (ECT), light therapy, and medications. These can be effective interventions for depression, especially when used in combination (Misri et al., 2000; Nulman, 2003; Rabheru, 2001; Spinelli & Endicott, 2003; Stamp, Williams, & Crowther, 1995). The various treatment options have the potential to reduce harmful effects to mother and child; therefore, it is essential for researchers to conduct meaningful investigations of the health determinants and risk factors associated with antenatal depression. This will help us to identify women with depression earlier so that they can receive the care that they need to reduce potential harm to the fetus and the mother. The research is increasing our knowledge about depression in pregnancy; however, there is much to learn about depression in pregnant women.

THE FEELINGS IN PREGNANCY AND MOTHERHOOD STUDY

The Feelings in Pregnancy and Motherhood Study investigated depression in 402 pregnant women enrolled in either the Healthy Mother Healthy Baby Program of the Saskatoon Health Region or the Westside Clinic of the Saskatoon Community Clinic, both located in Saskatoon, Canada. Women were invited to participate in the study at their first prenatal visit to either of the programs. Staff, clients, and management of the two programs were involved in the study design, questionnaire development, and data collection for this research project.

Healthy Mother Healthy Baby is a prenatal program designed to meet the needs of "hard to reach" pregnant women who are unlikely to access other prenatal services. The program strives to promote optimal pregnancy outcomes and healthy lifestyle choices by providing support and education to approximately 500 women a year. While the program was originally intended for Aboriginal women, new immigrants and refugees and teen mothers are also served by the program now. About 65 percent of women in the Healthy Mother Healthy Baby program are either First Nations or Métis, but all women who are socially at risk, including pregnant women who are attending high school or educational upgrade programs in the area, are invited to attend.

Healthy Mother Healthy Baby offers community-level interventions that focus on social and financial stressors during pregnancy. Women receive a broad range of services, including free prenatal vitamins, iron, Lactaid, milk coupons, and assistance with transportation to medical visits and prenatal classes. The program provides a variety of prenatal classes, such as single-parent classes, expert information (for example, legal), and special hospital tours for immigrant women. Women are followed throughout their pregnancies, through home or school visits. Every woman gets at least one postpartum visit in the first few weeks after the baby is born. Women with ongoing needs are referred to other community agencies before being discharged from the program (Bowen, 2003).

The Westside Clinic is part of the Saskatoon Community Clinic. The Saskatoon Community Clinic is a health care co-operative founded in 1962 (Saskatoon Community Clinic, 2004). It is a separate storefront clinic situated in an inner-city area of Saskatoon. This location is convenient for drop-in visits and is easily accessible by public transit. Women who attend the clinic experience extreme socio-economic stressors and often struggle with addiction problems that put their health and the health of their babies in peril. Westside Clinic provides medical care and psychosocial support to 60–80 pregnant women a year. All women who attend the clinic are encouraged to participate in the Healthy Mother Healthy Baby Program, but some women are struggling with addiction and other social problems that put them at very high risk and often they choose not to engage in any formal programming. The clinic offers drop-in prenatal clinics, which are open every Thursday afternoon.

Staff at Healthy Mother Healthy Baby had participated in other research studies. In their experience, women in the program and their partners were becoming increasingly suspicious of strangers coming into their homes to collect information. This was especially true when the information was of a personal nature, such as the extent of working hours outside the home, family violence, substance abuse, or any issues that they feared might be reported to authorities, and which could lead to problems with social services (for example, apprehension of the baby). Consequently, the manager and staff believed that they would be more successful in recruitment and data gathering than outside researchers would be.

The same philosophy exists about data collection for research purposes at the Westside Clinic. We offered to be present to collect the data at each of their regular weekly prenatal clinics, but instead, like Healthy Mother Healthy Baby, the clinic chose to recruit women directly and to collect the data themselves. Therefore, the principal investigator met regularly with the staff at both sites over many months to incorporate data collection into the different intake tools used by the staff at both sites. Since there was no remuneration available for data collection—for the women's participation in the study or other study activities—the principal investigator attempted to keep the study questions and changes to intake tools to a minimum.

This study involved the potential identification of women who might be depressed and/or have self-harm thoughts. Therefore, to prepare for their involvement in the study, a four-hour in-service was developed and presented to all staff both by the principal investigator and by a nurse therapist who specializes in anxiety and mood disorders, particularly postpartum depression. The in-service included information about the signs and symptoms, aetiology, effects, and treatment of antenatal depression, and how to manage client issues that might arise from any of the items on the study tools (for example, identification of self-harm thoughts). We developed a flow chart to describe what they would do in the event of an emergency. We also included information and instructions on administration and scoring of the depression screen used in the study.

The Edinburgh Postnatal Depression Scale (EPDS) is used to screen for depression in postnatal women, but was validated for use in pregnant women shortly after it was developed (Murray & Cox, 1990). The EPDS was chosen for the study because of its ease of use, extensive validation in different populations of women, including pregnant women (Cox & Holden, 2003), non-commercial availability, and the desire of both programs for an ongoing process for screening following their involvement in the study. The scale is meant to be self-administered. It includes ten items, each measured on a Likert scale. Each set of responses is scored from 0–3, to a maximum score of 30. The tool takes around five minutes to complete and score. As the title of the EPDS contains the term "depression," to avoid any potential bias of the woman's responses it was renamed "Feelings in Pregnancy and Motherhood" for use in this study.

Healthy Mother Healthy Baby staff also wanted to have information about depression and other emotions encountered by pregnant women to give to their clients. A booklet called "Feelings in Pregnancy and Motherhood" was developed for the women and their families. The staff edited and approved the content and the style of the booklet. It was available for all potential participants, whether they chose to join the study or not, and it is presently in use by program staff and other prenatal programs in the province.

We attended staff meetings, visited both offices, and kept in touch with the programs via telephone and email contact throughout the study. To ensure that the data collection tools addressed the unique circumstances and met the needs of this vulnerable population of women, we incorporated our theoretical perspectives into our study tools.

THEORETICAL PERSPECTIVES

Prenatal and obstetrical care has usually followed the biomedical model of assessments and interventions that focuses primarily on the physical well-being of the mother and the baby. This approach focuses on fixing or treating signs and symptoms of physical breakdown or disorder, with an emphasis on parameters such as weight gain, blood pressure, and fetal heart rate instead of extending the examination to the conditions and contexts in a woman's life that may give rise to these signs and symptoms. The population health approach, on the other hand, examines not just whether a woman is in need of immediate and expert physical care and treatment, but what factors in the family, social milieu, neighbourhoods, communities, and society at large contributed to the physical and mental symptoms treated in biomedical settings.

The population health approach to inquiry (formulation of questions, data collection, and interpretation) has the potential to increase knowledge about the prevalence and health determinants associated with antenatal depression. This will further our ability to promote levels of prevention through a more comprehensive approach to research on depression in pregnancy. The population health promotion prevention model for prenatal research we propose recognizes health determining factors at different social levels, and accordingly, there are different levels at which prevention and intervention is possible, such as at the level of the individual mother or pregnancy, family, community, institutions, systems, and society.

Population Health and Maternal Mental Health

While disease prevention has customarily focused on individuals, a population health approach is a more suitable framework for primary prevention within the community (Shah, 2003). The purpose of population health is not only to improve and maintain the health of the population, but also to decrease the inequities in health status among different groups of people and to improve the quality of life, for the population as a whole, over the lifespan (Shah, 2003). Population health requires significant attention to multiple determinants of health (Kindig & Stoddart, 2003). These multiple factors influence health beyond the usual health services and illness. Health determinants expand the scope of assessment to include a person's social, economic, and other life circumstances (WHO, 2007). The determinants that have previously been used to try to explain women's susceptibility to depression include: biology/genetics, environment, psychological disposition, and socio-economic status (Muramaki, 2002). However, with pregnancy, there may be hormonal changes that impact a woman's physical and mental health status. The World Health Organization states that identification and modification of the social factors that influence women's mental health offer the possibility of primary prevention of depression and, therefore, enduring positive changes in women's lives (WHO, 2004).

A population health approach to depression research and services focuses attention on root causes (for example, poverty, social disengagement) and solutions, increasing our understanding of the determinants of health associated with depression. A population health approach includes policies and strategies that deal with the wider influences of social inequalities, such as income (mal)distribution and lack of education, on health. The practices based on a population health perspective may have a stronger impact on health than those relying on the usual biomedical approaches, which have traditionally had a narrower focus on the health of the individual through means like changing unhealthy behaviours and attending treatment (Public Health Agency of Canada, 2001).

There are several levels of influence or determinants of health: the environment, the community, the family, the mother, the intrauterine environment, and the genetic makeup of the fetus all play a role. Population health perspectives guided this study in particular through guiding the conceptualization of broad categories of health determinants (for example, sociodemographic, obstetrical/biological, psychological, and behavioural) for socially vulnerable women. These health determinants work together at multiple levels and settings to affect the health status of the mother, and consequently, the well-being of the fetus and child.

Population health is a fitting approach to the study of depression during pregnancy, but the literature offers a mixed, and sometimes contradictory, account of the factors associated with antenatal depression. In the population health model for prenatal care that we have designed (shown in Figure 1), it is recognized that, from conception, the growing fetus is developing within the bounds of the genetic material endowed, but is invariably shaped and moulded by the environment within the womb and then the family. The fetus's initial determinants of health are largely influenced by its mother's health status. The determinants of prenatal health are affected by the mother's genetics/biology, life experiences, health history, and opportunities for healthy living. Some of these are at the individual level, while others are at the community, family, and societal levels.

Population health also increased our understanding of the lives and social conditions of the women we were hoping to recruit to the study and, therefore, broadened our scope in identifying the health determinants to be explored in the study. Jolene, the young mother, may not have easy access to medical facilities in her neighbourhood, which may have a negative effect on her ability to get adequate prenatal care and decrease the chances for detecting problems such as depression, and which may lead to less than optimal pregnancy outcomes. While these health service determinants are important to the health of the mother and the fetus, they were not within the scope of this initial study of antenatal depression.

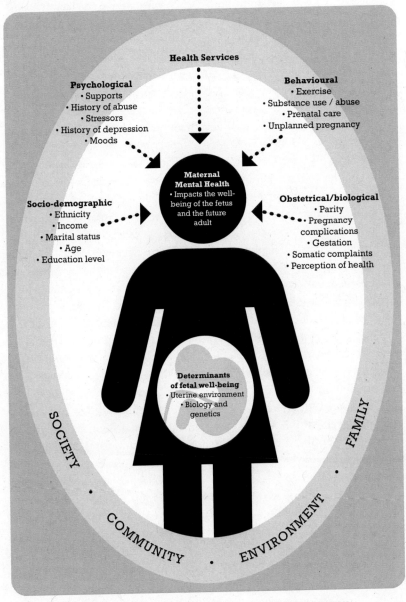

FIGURE 1. HEALTH DETERMINANTS AND ANTENATAL DEPRESSION

Levels of Prevention

Epidemiologic studies, such as this one, focusing on subpopulations, can help us to identify factors that put people at risk for disease (Gordis, 2004). There are three levels of prevention to consider: primary, secondary, and tertiary (Gordis, 2004). The goal of primary prevention is to identify risk factors for a disease before it has occurred, and to intervene on these risk factors to prevent the disease from occurring (Gordis, 2004). Primary prevention is the essence of community health practice: It enhances quality of life, and decreases morbidity, mortality, and overall health care costs (Shah, 2003).

Secondary prevention identifies those people who already have disease or precursors of disease or conditions. Secondary prevention can prevent mortality and complications of the disease through early detection (for example, screening), intervention, and treatment. Interventions that have focused on modifying these risk factors include prevention on both a primary and a secondary level (Gordis, 2004). Tertiary prevention often occurs after the disease has occurred and has had an impact on the person's level of health. It includes interventions that attempt to minimize the impact on quality of life and function, such as rehabilitation and reduction of sequelae, with a goal to help the person attain a new level of wellness; it also includes ongoing detection (Shah, 2003; Gordis, 2004).

The model shown in Figure 2, similar to Figure 1, recognizes that the fetus is nurtured directly within the intrauterine environment of the mother, developing its own biology with the genetic endowment it has received from both parents, under the influence of its mother's health status. The model proposes that primary, secondary, and tertiary prevention of antenatal depression at the maternal level will, in turn, exert primary prevention of the effects of antenatal depression in the fetus. All of the levels of prevention work collectively to improve the chances for optimal health of the developing fetus, which will, in turn, promote healthy outcomes into adulthood.

Within our model, the levels of prevention are experienced at the maternal and fetal level. At the maternal level, primary and secondary prevention involves universal screening and identification of antenatal depression. If women are found to be depressed they receive appropriate and timely treatment to reduce the depression. Secondary prevention of antenatal depression may also prevent the effects of antenatal depression, such as complications of pregnancy that affect both the mother and the fetus (for example, preterm delivery) (Chung et al., 2001) and worsening depression in the mother (Blazer, 1999; Heron et al., 2004).

Tertiary prevention involves policy and programming that promotes ongoing screening and accessible treatment of antenatal depression to improve the mental health of the mother. It involves interventions that lead to a policy and programs that promote the identification of, treatment for, and rehabilitation from antenatal depression. At a societal level, tertiary prevention focuses on the inequities in health determinants (socio-demographic, obstetrical/biological, psychological, and behavioural) that contribute to antenatal depression at individual, cultural, and community levels (Gordis, 2004).

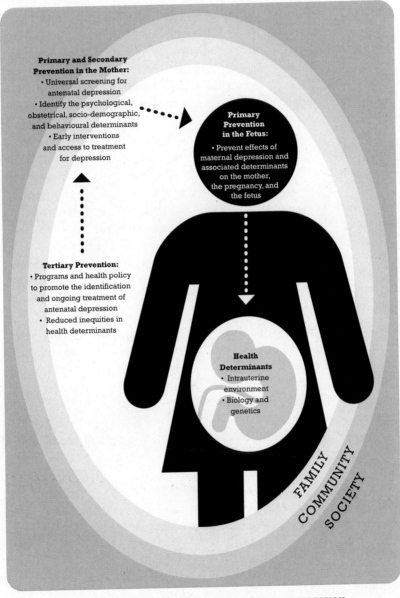

Primary and Secondary Prevention in the Mother:
• Universal screening for antenatal depression
• Identify the psychological, obstetrical, socio-demographic, and behavioural determinants
• Early interventions and access to treatment for depression

Primary Prevention in the Fetus:
• Prevent effects of maternal depression and associated determinants on the mother, the pregnancy, and the fetus

Tertiary Prevention:
• Programs and health policy to promote the identification and ongoing treatment of antenatal depression
• Reduced inequities in health determinants

Health Determinants
• Intrauterine environment
• Biology and genetics

FAMILY
COMMUNITY
SOCIETY

FIGURE 2. LEVELS OF PREVENTION FOR ANTENATAL DEPRESSION

With primary, secondary, and tertiary prevention occurring at the maternal level, primary prevention for the fetus should also follow. As conceptualized in this model in Figure 2, primary prevention for the fetus involves prevention of antenatal depression through the identification of risk factors in the mother. If the mother is depressed, prevention of the effects of antenatal depression on the fetus is critical, while also identifying the health determinants that put the mother at risk for developing antenatal depression. This knowledge can help us in targeting interventions that will promote the early identification of women with mental health and stress problems before they start to have children.

Integrated Model of Prevention and Population Health

Figure 3 shows our integrated model, which brings together the levels of prevention and the determinants of health perspectives into a comprehensive approach for prevention and population health promotion for research and action for pregnant women. The model has guided research activities, but also has stimulated action with prevention activities on all three levels. For instance, the model has guided knowledge translation activities that have promoted primary and secondary prevention through increased awareness of antenatal depression among local caregivers, the public, and professional groups.

The integrated model has led to the development of a Maternal Mental Health Program within a primary health care setting, which also houses the Healthy Mother Healthy Baby program (Bowen et al., 2008). The program provides primary prevention through public and professional education and individual pre-pregnancy consultations. Specialist practitioners provide evidence-based secondary and tertiary prevention to individuals and groups of women. The Maternal Mental Health Advisory Committee, which informs the program, includes women who have experienced depression in pregnancy, so that they can advise on depression health promotion and awareness initiatives. An evaluation of the effectiveness of the Maternal Mental Health Program is under way.

Finally, this integrated model has promoted secondary prevention of depression, which has led to the implementation of screening at some individual doctors' offices, within the Healthy Mother Healthy Baby Program, and at the Westside Clinic. It has also exerted tertiary prevention to inform public policy with the anticipated addition of depression screening to the recently revised provincial prenatal assessment form.

DISCUSSION

Our involvement of staff in the study design and recruitment of women has included education about depression and development of a process to get help for women who were identified as at risk for depression through the study questionnaire. The model has provided staff with increased knowledge and skills to be able to screen and identify women who are at increased vulnerability for depression, as well as a process to access emergency support and expert care.

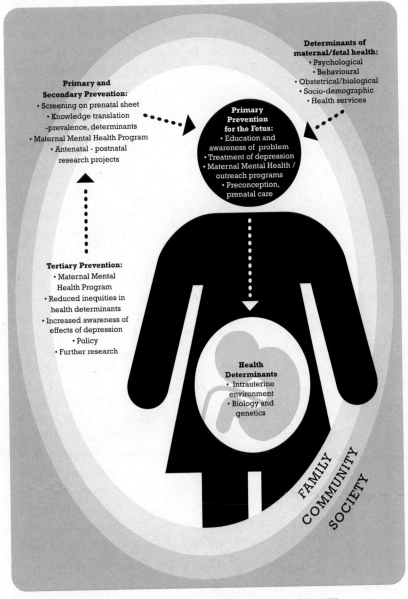

FIGURE 3. AN INTEGRATED MODEL OF POPULATION HEALTH
AND PREVENTION FOR ANTENATAL DEPRESSION

For Jolene, the single and pregnant mother of two, we now know that her high levels of stress, lack of support, and previous problems increase the likelihood that she may experience anxiety and depression. Her caregivers are now more cognizant of the signs and symptoms of depression and its potential impact on her health. They have a tool they can use to screen for depression and have a procedure to use to better support her in getting help for mental health problems. The staff at Healthy Mother Healthy Baby and the Westside Clinic care for women like Jolene all the time; their increased awareness and sensitivity to depression will position them to incorporate primary, secondary, and tertiary prevention and to continue to advocate for the women with respect to their mental health, while at the same time providing primary prevention for the fetus.

As we have identified, women living in socially high-risk situations are at increased risk for depression. However, because pregnancy is a time usually associated with joy and anticipation, the women themselves may not identify their feelings as depression. Therefore, it is essential to educate women and those who support them about the signs and symptoms associated with depression in pregnancy. The handout we have created for this purpose is very easy to read and has been well-received by women and staff.

We continue to use this integrated model to guide research on antenatal depression, its prevention, and its effects. We received funding from the Canadian Institutes of Health Research and extended the study so that we may compare the health determinants of depression in pregnancy and postpartum in this group of socially vulnerable women to the general population of women in our region. We have continued to refine the questionnaires and have provided much information to local physician offices and other caregivers.

CONCLUSION

We report here that a population health approach can successfully guide study design, data collection, and interpretation of the findings. It can help caregivers to identify the unique socio-demographic, obstetrical/biological, psychological, and behavioural determinants of health that put women at further risk better than the usual medical approach to either pregnancy or depression alone. The model increased our knowledge and understanding of the prevalence and determinants associated with antenatal depression in women in our community. We have promoted maternal mental health and resulting fetal well-being through all levels of prevention, screening, and care of women with antenatal depression at the primary, secondary, and tertiary levels of prevention.

Barker's theory of the origins of disease has renewed hope for improving the lives of individuals through greater understanding of the influences on fetal health (Barker, 1995) and, thereby, enriched the health of the population as a whole. Accordingly, the "Feelings in Pregnancy and Motherhood Study" was guided by the premise and hope that by learning more about the health determinants associated with depression in pregnancy, our further study would support using the levels of prevention previously defined and, subsequently, make a difference in the lives of mothers and their children. By incorporating a population health promotion and prevention approach, we have increased the scope of our study to identify a wide range of health determinants associated with antenatal depression and to use this information to promote prevention of maternal depression and, most importantly, to increase primary prevention for fetal health and well-being within the community.

This integrated model of antenatal depression inquiry and action, with its guiding principles of prevention and population health, has provided a framework for the identification of risk factors for depression in pregnancy and subsequent data collection and analysis. The model continues to direct our research and practice activities to improve the health status of vulnerable pregnant women, their unborn children, and their families.

Acknowledgements
We extend our gratitude to the women and staff at Healthy Mother Healthy Baby, Saskatoon Health Region and Westside Clinic, Saskatoon Community Clinic, Saskatoon, SK.

Funding
The study was supported by the Canadian Institutes of Health Research (CIHR, Grant 145179 Nazeem Muhajarine and Angela Bowen, co-principal investigators), the Community-University Institutes of Social Research (CUISR), and the CIHR-funded Community and Population Health Research (CPHR) Strategic Training Program within the Saskatchewan Population Health and Evaluation Research Unit (SPHERU) at the University of Saskatchewan.

The projects resulting from this study are supported through the Royal University Hospital Foundation, Saskatoon, SK, and the RBC Community Development Fund in conjunction with the College of Nursing, Saskatoon, SK. The evaluation of the Maternal Mental Health Program is funded by the Saskatchewan Health Research Foundation (SHRF)/Nursing Care Partnership.

REFERENCES

American Psychiatric Association. (2000). *Handbook of psychiatric measures* (1st ed.). Washington, DC: American Psychiatric Association.

Barker, D. J. P. (1995). The foetal origins of adult disease. *Biological Science, 262,* 37–43.

Blazer, D. G. (1999). Mood disorders: Epidemiology. In B. J. Sadock & V. A. Sadock (Eds.), *Comprehensive textbook of psychiatry* (Vol. 1, pp. 1298–1308). Philadelphia: Lippincott Williams & Wilkins.

Bonari, L., Bennett, H., Einarson, A., & Koren, G. (2004). Risks of untreated depression during pregnancy. *Canadian Family Physician.* Retrieved from http://www.cfpc.ca/cfp/2004/Jan/vo150-Jan-clinical-1.ASP February 6, 2005.

Bowen, A. (2003). Healthy Mother Healthy Baby. Retrieved from Community—University Institute for Social Research: http://www.usask.ca/cuisr/docs/pub_doc/health/Bowen.pdf

Bowen, A., Baetz, M., McKee, N., & Klebaum, N. (2008). Optimizing maternal mental health within a primary health care centre: a model program. *Canadian Journal of Community Mental Health, 27*(2), 105–116.

Bowen, A., & Muhajarine, N. (2006). Prevalence of depressive symptoms in an antenatal outreach program in Canada. *Journal of Obstetric, Gynecologic, and Neonatal Nursing, 35*(4), 492–498.

Bowen, A., Stewart, N., Baetz, M., & Muhajarine, N. (2009). Antenatal depression in socially high-risk women in Canada. *Journal of Epidemiology and Community Health, 63,* 414–416. doi:10.1136/jech.2008.078832

Caplan, H. L., Cogill, S. R., Alexandra, H., Robson, K. M., Katz, R., & Kumar, R. (1989). Maternal depression and the emotional development of the child. *British Journal of Psychiatry, 154,* 818–822.

Chung, T. K. H., Lau, K., Yip, A. S. K., Chiu, H. F. K., & Lee, D. T. S. (2001). Antepartum depressive symptomatology is associated with adverse obstetric and neonatal outcomes. *Psychosomatic Medicine, 63*(5), 830–834.

Cole, B., Kane, C., Killeen, M., Mohr, W., Nield-Anderson, L., & Kurlowicz, L. (2000, April). *Responding to The Global Burden of Disease* [White paper]. Accessed from the International Society of Psychiatric-Mental Health Nurses: http://www.ispn-psych.org/docs/4-00Global-Burden.pdf

Cox, J. L., & Holden J. M. (2003). *Perinatal mental health: A guide to the Edinburgh Postnatal Depression Scale.* Glasgow, UK: Bell & Bain Ltd. ·

Field, T. (1997). The treatment of depressed mothers and their infants. In L. Murray & P.J. Cooper (Eds.), *Postpartum depression and child development.* New York: Guilford Press.

Glover, V., & O'Connor, T. G. (2002). Effects of antenatal stress and anxiety: Implications for development and psychiatry. *British Journal of Psychiatry, 180,* 389–391.

Goodman, J. H. (2004). Paternal postpartum depression, its relationship to maternal postpartum depression, and its implications for family health. *Journal of Advanced Nursing, 45*(1), 26–35.

Gordis, L. (2004). *Epidemiology* (3rd ed.). Philadelphia: Elsevier Saunders.

Hellin, D., & Waller, G. (1992). Mother's mood and infant feeding: Prediction of problems and practices. *Journal of Reproductive and Infant Psychology, 10,* 39–51.

Heron, J., O'Connor, T. G., Evans, J., Golding, J., & Glover, V. (2004). The course of anxiety and depression through pregnancy and the postpartum in a community sample. *Journal of Affective Disorders, 80*(1), 65–73.

Kahn, R. S., Certain, L., & Whitaker, R. C. (2002). A re-examination of smoking before, during, and after pregnancy. *American Journal of Public Health, 92*(11), 1801–1808.

Kindig, D., & Stoddart, G. (2003). What is population health? *American Journal of Public Health 93*(3), 380–383.

Maki, P., Veijola, J., Rasanen, P., Joukamaa, M., Valonen, P., & Jokelainen, J., et al. (2003). Criminality in the offspring of antenatally depressed mothers: a 33-year follow-up of the Northern Finland 1966 Birth Cohort. *Journal of Affective Disorders, 74,* 273–278.

Marcus, S. M., Flynn, H. A., Blow, F.C., & Barry, K. L. (2003). Depressive symptoms among pregnant women screened in obstetrics settings. *Journal of Women's Health, 12*(4), 373–380.

Mathers, C.D., Bernard, C., Moesgaard-Iburg, K., Inoue, M., Fat, D., Shibuya, K., Stein C., Tomijima N., & Xu, H. (2002). Global Burden of Disease in 2002: Data sources, methods and results. *Health Statistics and Health Information Systems.* Retrieved from World Health Organization: http://www.who.int/healthinfo/paper54.pdf

Misri, S., Dim, J., Riggs, K. W., & Kostaras, X. (2000). Paroxetine levels in postpartum depressed women, breast milk, and infant serum. *Journal of Clinical Psychiatry, 61*(11), 828–832.

Muramaki, J. (2002). Gender and depression: Explaining the different rates of depression between men and women. *Perspectives in Psychology,* 27–34.

Murray, D., & Cox, J. (1990). Screening for depression during pregnancy with the Edinburgh Depression Scale (EPDS). *Journal of Reproductive and Infant Psychology, 8,* 99–107.

Murray L., & Cooper, P. J. (2003). Intergenerational transmission of affective and cognitive processes associated with depression: Infancy and the pre-school years. In I. M. Goodyer (Ed.), *Unipolar depression: A lifetime perspective* (pp. 17–42). Oxford: Oxford University Press.

Murray L., Cooper P. J., & Hipwell, A. (2003). Mental health of parents caring for infants. *Archives of Women's Mental Health, 6*(Suppl. 2), 71–77.

Norbeck, J. S., & Tilden, V. P. (1983). Life stress, social support, and emotional disequilibrium in complications of pregnancy: A prospective, multivariate study. *Journal of Health and Social Behaviour, 24,* 30–46.

Nulman, I. (2003). Child development following exposure to tricyclic antidepressants or fluoxetine throughout fetal life: A prospective controlled study. *American Journal of Psychiatry, 159,* 1889–1895.

O'Connor, T. G., Heron, J., Glover, V., & The Alspac Study Team. (2002). Antenatal anxiety predicts child behavioral/emotional problems independently of postnatal depression. *Journal of the American Academy of Child & Adolescent Psychiatry, 41*(12), 1470–1477.

Public Health Agency of Canada. (2001). *The Population Health Template Working Tool, 2005.* Retrieved from http://www.phac-aspc.gc.ca/ph-sp/phdd/pdf/template_tool.pdf

Rabheru, K. (2001). The use of electroconvulsive therapy in special patient populations. *Canadian Journal of Psychiatry, 46*(8), 710–719.

Saskatoon Community Clinic (2004). About us. Retrieved from http://www.saskatooncommunityclinic.ca/about_us.htm February 6, 2005.

Seto, M., Cornelius, M. D., Goldschmidt, L., Morimoto, K., & Day, N. L. (2005). Long-term effects of chronic depressive symptoms among low-income childrearing mothers. *Maternal & Child Health Journal, 9*(3), 263–271.

Shah, C. P. (2003). *Public health and preventative medicine in Canada* (5th ed.). Toronto: Elsevier Canada.

Spinelli, M. G., & Endicott J. (2003). Controlled clinical trial of interpersonal psychotherapy versus parenting education program for depressed pregnant women. *American Journal Psychiatry, 160*(3), 555–562.

Spirito, A., Ruggiero, L., Coustan, D., McGarvey, S., & Bond, A. (1992). Mood state of women with diabetes during pregnancy. *Journal of Reproductive and Infant Psychiatry, 10*, 29–38.

Stamp, G. E., Williams, A. S., & Crowther, C. A. (1995). Evaluation of antenatal and postnatal support to overcome postnatal depression: A randomized, controlled trial. *Birth, 22*(3), 138–143.

WHO (World Health Organization). (2004). Prevention of Mental Disorders. Effective interventions and policy options. *Mental Health Evidence and Research (MER)*. Retrieved from http://www.who.int/mental_health/evidence/en/prevention_of_mental_disorders_sr. pdf January 29, 2005.

WHO (World Health Organization). (2006). Women's Mental Health: A Public Health Concern. *Regional Health Forum: WHO South-East Asia Region, 5*(1). Retrieved from http://searo.who.int/EN/Section1243/Section1310/Section1343/Section1344/Section1353_5282.htm December 12, 2006.

WHO (World Health Organization). (2007). The Determinants of Health. *Health Impact Assessment (HIA)*. Retrieved from http://www.who.int/hia/evidence/doh/en/ October 31, 2007.

Wilkerson, D. S., Volpe, A. G., Dean, R. S., & Titus, J. B. (2002). Perinatal complications as predictors of infantile autism. *International Journal of Neuroscience, 9*(112), 1085–1098.

Zuckerman, B., Bauchner, H., Parker, S., & Cabral, H. (1990). Maternal depressive symptoms during pregnancy and newborn irritability. *Journal of Developmental and Behavioural Pediatrics, 11*(4), 190–194.

Zuckerman, B. S., Amaro, H., Bauchner, H., & Cabral, H. (1989). Depression symptoms during pregnancy: Relationship to poor health behaviors. *American Journal of Obstetrics and Gynecology, 160*(5), 1107–1111.

The Cousin of Globalization:
Neo-liberalism and Child-Relevant Policy

Jennifer Cushon and Nazeem Muhajarine

INTRODUCTION

Globalization is a broad, complex, and often contested concept. Most simply, globalization refers to the various processes that intensify the interdependence of people, businesses, and countries through increased economic integration and advances in communications technology (Labonte & Torgerson, 2005). It is widely acknowledged that since the 1980s the processes of globalization have been a defining force for every corner of the globe in terms of politics, social lives, economics, the environment, culture, and technology (McBride, 2005). The political economic theory of neo-liberalism has facilitated the processes of globalization over the past three decades in Canada and elsewhere. Neo-liberalism has been referred to as the "cousin" of globalization (Keil, 2002). Neo-liberalism "proposes that human well-being can best be advanced by liberating individual entrepreneurial freedoms and skills within an institutional framework characterized by strong private property rights, free markets, and free trade" (Harvey, 2005, p. 2).

In the globalization literature, an expanding area of interest has been the health-related impacts of globalization. However, within this literature there is a lack of evidence regarding Canadian policy responses to the changing contexts for health that have resulted due to the rise of the twin concepts: globalization and neo-liberalism. Moreover, despite the growing acknowledgement that globalization profoundly shapes and dictates economic and social policy, there is a paucity of literature related to globalization and its impact on domestic policy in Canada. In response to some of these gaps in the literature, a mixed methods case study was undertaken to investigate the political and economic pathways by which globalization impacts the determinants of health and health outcomes in a mid-sized Canadian city (Saskatoon, Saskatchewan), focusing specifically on low-income children. This paper presents results from one component of the case study: an environmental scan of federal, provincial, and municipal policy that has direct relevance for the health of low-income children in Saskatoon.

NEO-LIBERALISM, CANADIAN POLICY, AND CHILD HEALTH: DEFINING TERMS AND SETTING THE CONTEXT

As a political economic theory, neo-liberalism has its foundation in eighteenth-century liberalism, which was premised on two central assumptions: the first assumption is that the exercise of individual self-interest will lead to the greatest good for the greatest number; the second, that the market will ensure optimal benefits for everyone. In the post–World War II era, the political philosophy of liberalism began to change due to attempts to compensate for the failings of the market through the building of the Keynesian welfare state. Neo-liberalism, as practiced today, harkens back to old precepts of eighteenth-century liberalism, emphasizing the primacy of the market, liberalization, deregulation, privatization, and the importance of personal responsibility. Not surprisingly, a retrenchment of the welfare state often occurs under neo-liberal governments, particularly in areas of social welfare (Smith, 2002; Teeple, 2000).

In Canada, the shift towards a neo-liberal orientation is often dated to 1985, when the final report of the Macdonald Commission, also known as the Royal Commission on the Economic Union and Development Prospects for Canada, was released (Inwood, 2005). The Macdonald Commission restated a confidence in the market to efficiently and effectively allocate resources for the well-being of Canadians (Fudge & Cossman, 2002). Canada's shift towards a neo-liberal state was catalyzed due to a number of factors, including the economic crisis of 1981–1982; a large debt; the liberalization of trade on a more global scale; the increasing strength of Canada's capitalist class; and the rise of neo-liberal governments in the United States and Britain (Inwood, 2005; McBride, 2005).

Neo-liberalism was further entrenched in Canada and its provinces in the 1990s. The federal and provincial governments became preoccupied by certain policy considerations such as:

- trade liberalization was to be the dominant economic development strategy, while the welfare state had to be reconfigured to fit this competitive stance;

- large deficits were to be avoided; and
- tax reforms and tax cuts had to be enacted to further the competitive trade environment and to allay fears that government spending was out of control (Brown, 2002).

These policy considerations have continued to dominate Canadian public policy to this day.

Neo-liberalism has exacerbated tensions in Canada's federal system of governance. The domestic tendency has been to decentralize power to the provinces, but neo-liberalism and international competitiveness concerns tend to encourage federal government involvement. Through its budgetary powers, the federal government still has a fair amount of sway in terms of policy across the country (McBride, 2005). Some provinces, such as Ontario and Alberta, have not supported the federal government's continued and sustained involvement in economic policy (Brown, 2002; Ruggeri, 2005). Areas of social concern have been largely devolved to the provinces. Devolution of power was partly driven by the Quebec referendum and the belief that devolution in certain policy domains would quell the calls for separation (McBride, 2005). Since the provinces are now mainly responsible for social policy, the policies implemented that have direct relevance for children and their health may vary greatly from province to province. Thus, this environmental scan and its findings are specific to the provincial context of Saskatchewan, although they may hold lessons for other provinces with similar policies.

But why should we be concerned with neo-liberal policies from a population health standpoint? First, the adoption of neo-liberal policies in governments throughout the world has led to a gradual (in some cases rapid) dismantling of the welfare state (Tanzi, 2006). The retrenchment of the welfare state in many countries, including Canada, has the potential to fundamentally and negatively affect child health. A strong welfare state, with higher levels of social expenditure and taxation to support it, is important for the health and development of populations. States with a strong commitment to welfare have longer life expectancy, lower maternal mortality, and fewer low birth weight infants (Coburn, 2000).

Neo-liberalism privileges the privatization not only of assets and economic production, but also of policy-making (Coburn, 2000; Fudge & Cossman, 2002; Hay, 2006). This has already occurred to some extent in Canada's federal system, with the devolution of social responsibility moving down from the federal system to the provinces and municipalities. At its most extreme, the privatization of policy-making means that certain areas of social development are privatized completely. Responsibility for social issues is then divested to the community or the individual (Hay, 2006). The devolution of responsibility for social development translates into fewer dollars spent on social programs such as child care or social housing.

Empirical studies have found that neo-liberal policies have the propensity to deepen poverty among populations that were already vulnerable to poverty (Wade, 2004). Studies have also demonstrated that neo-liberalism is highly correlated with increasing income inequality within and between countries (Coburn, 2000; Coburn, 2004; Cornia & Kiiski, 2001; Young, 2004). Income inequality has enormous health implications. For instance, Wilkinson (1992) has found that there is a strong association between life expectancy and income inequality within a country. The pathways by which income inequality results in poor health outcomes are not well-defined. However, one pathway may consist of income inequality leading to decreased levels of social cohesion in society, which in turn lowers health (Coburn, 2004; Wallerstein, 1992). The income and social status of families, including disparities in these measures, are considered critical determinants of health for infants and children.

POLICY-MAKING IN A GLOBALIZED ERA: AN ENVIRONMENTAL SCAN
This environmental scan encompassed policy from 1980 onwards, except where historical information was useful for providing greater context. Although the origins of globalization may date far back in history, the 1980s are marked as a turning point in the current conceptualization of globalization. This decade was witness to the downfall of socialism, rapid developments in information technology, and the wholesale adoption of neo-liberal policies by most national governments (Cornia, 2001; Teeple, 2000).

This environmental scan was limited to policies that specifically impact children from prenatal to age five. This period in child development is considered fundamental to later health and well-being (Canadian Population Health Initiative, 2006; Hertzman, 2000; Hertzman, 2004; Irwin, Siddiqi, & Hertzman, 2007). It is also important to define the age of the children who are being investigated since the effects of globalization can be age-dependent (Thompson, 2002). Low-income children were of particular interest since they are the most vulnerable to the negative consequences of globalization (Keating & Mustard, 1993).

In this environmental scan, five key policy areas were examined: early childhood policy, social welfare policy, education and child care policy, housing policy, and labour policy (that is, those labour policies that directly impact the family and children, such as parental benefits and leave). The overall case study was conducted from a population health perspective; thus, the findings in this environmental scan largely speak to the non-medical determinants of child health (Kindig & Stoddart, 2003). It is well-established that people's health is affected mainly by their social and economic situations. The most effective health-enhancing policy is one that increases investments in the social and economic circumstances of populations, rather than one that increases access to medical care for individuals (Low et al., 2005). The policies reviewed in this environmental scan were almost exclusively social and economic.

A number of databases and websites were searched for relevant policy documents. First, the Canadian Social Research Links—a website that contains an enormous amount of policy literature related to social services—was searched. Second, the Canadian Research Index (formerly Microlog) was searched using the following terms: housing, child welfare, poverty, parent benefits, child development, education, child care, employment insurance, public welfare, social policy, and welfare. Each of the aforementioned terms was entered with the geographic qualifiers of Saskatoon, Saskatchewan, and Canada. In addition, the websites of organizations such as Canadian Policy Research Networks, the National Council of Welfare, and the Organisation for Economic Cooperation and Development were searched for relevant publications.

Once articles and documents had been selected for relevance from websites and databases, they were scanned and placed into one of the five selected policy areas. Articles and documents were read and the relevant information was noted in a data template. The following section highlights the principal findings from the environmental scan and is organized according to the five policy areas mentioned above.

EARLY CHILDHOOD POLICY

Eradicating child poverty has been a stated policy priority of the federal and provincial governments in Canada since the 1980s. A seminal moment in Canadian child-relevant policy occurred in 1989 when Members of the House of Commons unanimously supported a resolution to end child poverty by the year 2000 (National Council of Welfare, Spring 1997). In response to this resolution, the federal and provincial governments engaged in a number of priority-setting exercises and enacted certain policy mechanisms. For example, following the 1990 World Summit for Children, the federal government created *Brighter Futures: Canada's Action Plan for Children*. The aim of this initiative was to ensure the effectiveness and coordination of activities related to children, across federal departments. Also as a result of the 1990 World Summit for Children, Health Canada expanded their children's programming in a number of areas, usually in the form of community-based interventions (Jenson & Thompson, 1999). Reacting to the federal government's *Action Plan for Children*, Saskatchewan introduced its own *Action Plan for Children* in 1993, to ensure greater coordination across provincial departments serving families and children (Government of Saskatchewan, 1999; Mahon, 2001).

The National Children's Agenda (NCA) was announced in the 1997 Speech from the Throne. The NCA discussed the implementation of a National Child Benefit (NCB), and this was formally introduced in 1998. The main policy mechanism used to combat child poverty in Canada has been child benefits. Tax deductions tend to disproportionately benefit higher income families, whereas a benefit is considered more beneficial for disadvantaged families (Baker, 1997). The NCB was premised upon the principle that families are best off when parents participate in the labour market (Federal, Provincial and Territorial Ministers Responsible for Social Services, 2007; Laurent & Vaillancourt, 2004).

The provinces and territories had the option of adjusting their own social assistance or child benefit payments equivalent to the National Child Benefit. This is commonly termed the NCB clawback (National Council of Welfare, 2008). The funds that result from this adjustment process can then be invested in new or enhanced programs that target low-income children (Federal, Provincial and Territorial Ministers Responsible for Social Services, 2007). Parents in the labour market are allowed to retain all of their NCB, whereas the clawback only applies to parents on social assistance (National Council of Welfare, 2008; Raphael, 2007). The NCB is not offered to families on social assistance in Saskatchewan. In Saskatchewan, the funds that have resulted from the NCB clawback have been used for a number of initiatives, such as programs aimed at housing and shelter allowances; nutrition in schools; child care costs for low-income working families; health benefits that target dental services, optometry, prescriptions, etc.; community school projects; and employment support/training (Federal, Provincial and Territorial Ministers Responsible for Social Services, 2007).

The federal government, the territories and nine of the provinces (Quebec chose to opt out) signed the Early Childhood Development initiative in 2000 in order to increase and expand provincial programs for young children and families. The funding provided through this initiative was to be used in four general areas: 1) the promotion of healthy pregnancy, birth, and infancy; 2) improving family functioning; 3) fostering better early childhood development, learning, and care; and 4) strengthening community supports (Federal, Provincial and Territorial Ministers Responsible for Social Services, 2007). The province of Saskatchewan committed to expanding early childhood development programs in the four areas selected by the federal government and reporting annually on progress and funds spent. A cornerstone of Saskatchewan's response to early childhood development has been the

KidsFirst Program. Introduced in 2001, the *KidsFirst* Program focuses on prevention and early intervention for children prenatal to age five. *KidsFirst* targets children who are considered vulnerable to social disadvantage (Government of Saskatchewan, n.d.).

SOCIAL WELFARE POLICY

Since 1966, the federal government paid for half of all social programs in the provinces through the Canadian Assistance Plan (CAP). Funding from CAP was directed towards social assistance, special care homes, child welfare, and other welfare services. Health services and education were financed under the Established Programs Financing (EPF) (Jenson & Thompson, 1999). In 1996, the Canada Health and Social Transfer (CHST) replaced CAP and EPF. The CHST provided block funding for health, post-secondary education, social assistance, and social services (Hunter & Miazdyck, 2003). In April 2004, the CHST was further split into two separate transfers: the Canada Health Transfer (CHT) for health care; and the Canada Social Transfer (CST) for education, social assistance, and social services (Human Resources and Social Development Canada, n.d.). The elimination of CAP led to large reductions in federal funding for social policy in the provinces (McBride, 2005; National Council of Welfare, Spring 1997).

Since the Canada Health and Social Transfer is a block-funded program, it allowed the provinces to experiment with welfare delivery. Across the country, this has led to variations on workfare, an approach to welfare that is based on the presupposition that individuals and families thrive most when they are part of the labour market (Hunter & Miazdyck, 2003). In Saskatchewan, when the New Democratic Party defeated the Progressive Conservative government in 1991, the new government criticized the previous government for paltry welfare rates, unfair controls, and treating people on welfare without dignity. Recommendations for change were acted upon in some instances (for example, the elimination of mandatory cheque pickup, indexed benefits, etc.), but these changes were largely reversed later in the 1990s when the CHST was introduced (Government of Saskatchewan, 1996).

In the summer of 1998, the Government of Saskatchewan unveiled its approach to workfare: the *Building Independence– Investing in Families* initiative. This initiative was composed of six programs, with three that were directly targeted at child poverty, including the Saskatchewan Employment Supplement (SES), a monthly grant paid to supplement income for low-income working families; the Saskatchewan Child Benefit (SCB), a monthly allowance paid to all low-income families with children; and the Family Health Benefit (FHB) for supplementary health benefits for low-income working families (Hunter

& Miazdyck, 2003). Following the introduction of workfare in Saskatchewan, the number of social assistance cases dropped precipitously. This decrease in caseloads has been attributed to fewer people qualifying for welfare, rather than the "good news" story of people leaving welfare for quality, paid employment (International Development Research Centre, n.d.).

A further change to social assistance in Saskatchewan occurred in 2003, when the government introduced the Transitional Employment Allowance (TEA). The regulations for TEA stated that it was directed at "persons in need who are participating in certain pre-employment programs" (Hunter & Donovan, 2005, p. 2) or those who would not require welfare in the long term. The TEA program was viewed by the government not as social assistance, but rather as a means for people to become independent and enter the workforce. TEA increased the already stringent eligibility requirements for social assistance that had been enforced under workfare. Many new applicants to social assistance are now placed on TEA for a short period of time. The TEA program tends to facilitate employment, albeit at the lowest end of the pay scale (Hunter & Miazdyck, 2003; Hunter & Donovan, 2005).

CHILD CARE AND EDUCATION POLICY

Unlike most developed countries, Canada does not have a national child care system (Foster & Broad, 1998). The Progressive Conservative federal government led by Brian Mulroney attempted to institute a national child care system, but the proposed program was not supported by child care advocates. The proposed program was quickly shelved (White, 2002). The federal government became involved in the policy area of child care again in 1993, when the Liberal government promised to expand child care (Laurent & Vaillancourt, 2004). After a decade of minimal action by the federal Liberals, a major commitment to early learning and child care was made in 2003, and the Multilateral Framework Agreement on Early Learning and Child Care was introduced (Government of Canada, 2004). Despite the federal government's intentions, the provincial/territorial governments were hesitant to enter into a multilateral agreement due to concerns about funding only being available to support principles set out by the federal government and for non-profit child care. Forgoing negotiations with all of the provinces and territories at one table, the federal government entered into bilateral agreements-in-principle with nine provinces, including Saskatchewan, between April and November 2005 (Cool, 2007).

When the Conservatives assumed federal leadership in January 2006, it was announced that the bilateral child care agreements with the provinces would be cancelled after one year. To replace the bilateral agreements, the federal government announced a $1200 per year Choice in Child Care Allowance for each child under the age of six. A Community Child Care Investment Program was also announced, which was intended to provide tax credits to employers that created new child care spaces. There was very little uptake of the Community Child Care Investment Program; therefore, in 2007, the federal government redirected the $250 million a year it had committed to the Community Child Care Investment Program to the provinces and territories to support the creation of child care spaces. In the 2007 budget, the federal government announced a 25 percent tax credit for businesses that created child care spaces (Cool, 2007).

Although there have been many failed attempts to create a national child care program in Canada, child care has mainly been a provincial responsibility. Provincial child care programs vary widely in terms of goals. All provinces provide subsidies for low-income parents, and most provinces require that child care services are regulated (White, 2002). Municipalities in Canada generally have no role, or a very circumscribed role, in terms of early childhood education and development (Doherty, Friendly, & Beach, 2003). Most provinces in Canada, such as Saskatchewan, offer some government monies for child care centres. But child care is essentially an enrolment-driven system, with programs largely dependent on parent fees (Foster & Broad, 1998). In Saskatchewan, the government has favoured non-profit provision, which has resulted in a publicly funded system that is privately delivered (Jenson & Thompson, 1999).

An important component of early childhood education is preschool programs (Kamerman et al., 2003). Preschool has never been publicly funded for all children in Saskatchewan. In 1997, Saskatchewan Education implemented a part-day preschool program that was publicly funded for children aged 3–4 who were considered to be at risk (Childcare Resource and Research Unit, 1998). Following preschool, the majority of Saskatchewan's young children enter into kindergarten, which has evolved into a system that targets five-year-olds in order to prepare them for entry into the formal school system (Doherty, Friendly, & Beach, 2003). Publicly funded kindergarten programs are operated in Saskatoon by both the Saskatoon Public School Division and the Saskatoon Catholic School Division (Muhajarine et al., 2007). In the 1990s, the Government of Saskatchewan cut the amount of grants to school boards and municipalities, which resulted in higher property taxes and user fees in the cities (Warnock, 2003).

HOUSING POLICY

Housing policy in Canada has been historically set by the federal government. Beginning in the 1970s, provincial governments began to play a more prominent role in this policy area. By the 1980s, housing policy was a shared responsibility between the federal and provincial governments. Canada had one of the most comprehensive social housing programs in the world until the mid-1980s. But this decade marked a turning point in federal housing policy, with large cuts to housing budgets and programs. By 1993, federal funding for housing had become nearly non-existent. In 1996, the federal government devolved all responsibility for housing to the provinces and territories (Carter & Polevychok, 2004).

Once housing responsibilities were devolved to the provinces, in most instances, the responsibility was moved further down (Cooper, 2001). In Saskatchewan, the Saskatchewan Housing Corporation (SHC) is responsible for managing the funds contributed by the municipal, provincial, and federal governments for affordable housing. In fact, SHC is responsible for managing only about 3 percent of its housing portfolio, with 60 percent being managed by housing authorities and about 37 percent being managed by non-profit groups. In Saskatoon, a large proportion of the SHC portfolio is managed by the Saskatoon Housing Authority (Government of Saskatchewan, 2005).

The City of Saskatoon's role in housing was not clearly defined until the release of the Housing Business Plan in 2006. The goals of this business plan were: affordability of housing, balanced growth/stability, safe and adequate housing, monitoring demographics, and meeting the need for innovative housing. The City of Saskatoon does offer some incentives for particular forms of development, such as residential housing projects for low-income families, incentives to build residential property downtown, and incentives to build in older, more impoverished neighbourhoods in the city (City of Saskatoon, 2006). However, there are also a number of municipal policies that discourage investment in affordable housing. Residential rental units are the most common form of housing for low-income households, but the City of Saskatoon has introduced tax policies that discourage building rental property. The municipal government taxes multi-residential buildings at a higher rate than residential housing. Federal government tax policies regarding capital gains also tend to penalize those who own or build rental property (Merriman & Pringle, 2008).

LABOUR POLICY

Since the 1980s, responsibility for the funding of Unemployment Insurance (UI) has been gradually shifted from the federal government to employers and employees. In 1990, the federal government's responsibilities for financing were completely eliminated and the entire cost of the fund was born by employers and employees (Lin, 1998). Changes in financing signalled a retrenchment of the UI system, which has continued unabated and has led to more stringent entrance requirements and reduced benefit rates (Lin, 1998; Maki, Friesen, & Siedule, 2001). With the passing of Bill C-12 in 1996, the UI system was renamed Employment Insurance (EI). Bill C-12 was in keeping with the 1995 federal budget, which pledged to reduce the costs of UI by 10 percent (Government of Canada, 1995). Under UI/EI restructuring, large segments of the population were not eligible for EI assistance due to more stringent eligibility requirements (Ismael, 2006).

A component of the UI/EI system that facilitates employment in the labour force, most often female employment, is parental leave policy (Kamerman et al., 2003). Responsibility for the administration of parental leave is shared between the federal government and the provincial/territorial governments. The restructuring of the UI/EI system in 1996 had major repercussions for parental leaves. Under the EI program, only those who had worked 700 hours in the previous 52 weeks were eligible for maternal or parental leave, which was double the number of hours that had been required prior to the introduction of EI. Due to these eligibility restrictions, less than half of all families with a newborn were eligible for a paid maternal or parental leave in 1998 (Jenson & Thompson, 1999). Those parents who do qualify for EI only receive 55 percent of their wages for up to one year, which is often not enough for most families to subsist on (McIntosh, Muhajarine, & Klatt, 2004).

Another labour policy instrument that has the potential to affect low-income families is the minimum wage (Saunders, 2005). Minimum wages are determined by each province/territory. Currently, an individual working full-time at minimum wage in Saskatchewan does not meet the Low-Income Cut-Off (LICO).[1] During the period 1991 to 2006 in Saskatchewan, the minimum wage increased by a total of $2.95. Yet, when this amount was reviewed in terms of purchasing power, it was found that the purchasing power of the minimum wage had declined steadily (Saskatchewan Minimum Wage Board, 2007). In October 2007, the Government of Saskatchewan announced its intentions to gradually raise the minimum wage to be more on par with the LICO (Government of Saskatchewan, 2008).

DISCUSSION

This environmental scan of federal, provincial, and municipal policies that have direct relevance for low-income children in Saskatoon, Saskatchewan, revealed a number of themes. First, there has been a gradual retrenchment of the welfare state in Canada, Saskatchewan, and Saskatoon. For instance, the elimination of the Canadian Assistance Plan was touted by the National Council of Welfare (1995) as, "the worst social policy initiative by the federal government in more than a generation" (p. 26). This declaration was based on the fact that the elimination of CAP led to large reductions in federal funding for health care, post-secondary education, social assistance, and social services in the provinces (National Council of Welfare, Spring 1997). With reduced federal funding, the Government of Saskatchewan completely overhauled its social assistance system and introduced workfare—a neo-liberal solution to poverty that emphasizes the importance of entering the market and taking personal responsibility. The restructuring of the UI/EI system has also had far-reaching implications for Canada's families. Ismael (2006) argues that the restructuring of UI/EI represented the dismantling of Canada's fundamental anti-poverty program.

Even though the retrenchment of the welfare state was witnessed in most policy areas covered in this environmental scan, there is one policy area that stands as an exception—early childhood development. Children have remained a policy priority of both the federal and provincial governments since the 1980s (Wiegers, 2002). In Saskatchewan, early childhood development policy has favoured targeted over universal approaches. In fact, across all of the provinces there has been a trend towards providing targeted programs for children considered "at risk" (Mahon, 2001). Means testing for social programs and services is also increasingly common. Targeting for program and service delivery signifies a retrenchment of the welfare state, although not on as grand a scale as in some other policy areas. There has also been a trend towards implementing community-based interventions for at-risk children. Although community-based interventions allow for the integration of local context into program planning and delivery, this represents a further shift away from government responsibility for social programming.

Canada's and Saskatchewan's sustained policy focus on early childhood development suggests that these jurisdictions have partially subscribed to a social investment strategy. The term "social investment state" was first coined by Anthony Giddens. Social investment states privilege entrepreneurship and those policies that encourage greater participation in the structures of society, such as the market. Under a social investment strategy, individualist solutions to societal issues are proposed. In addition, as suggested in the name, the social investment state is concerned with making investments in the future, particularly in childhood development (Saint-Martin, 2007). Further analysis, potentially in the form of content analysis, is required to determine how greatly the social investment strategy has influenced Canadian and Saskatchewan child-relevant policy.

Another theme to emerge was that the restructuring of public policy in Canada and Saskatchewan under neo-liberalism has encouraged the devolution of power/responsibility. Although the federal government retains power in the area of economic policy, responsibility for social policy has largely fallen on the shoulders of the provinces. However, increased responsibility for the provinces was accompanied by large reductions in the federal transfer of funds (Ruggeri, 2005). This has encouraged even further devolution to municipal governments and sometimes even further down to community-based organizations or to the individual. Municipal governments in Canada, such as the City of Saskatoon, have been saddled with more responsibilities, but they actually have very little policy-making clout and possibilities for revenue generation (Mahon, 2001; Sancton, 2002). So, while cities represent "the locus of productive economic activities and hope for the future" (Stren & Polese, 2000, p. 11) in a globalized economy, they actually have very little room to manoeuvre when addressing the impacts of globalization and neo-liberalism within their communities.

Despite the decentralizing-centralizing tensions in the federal system that have been exacerbated by the processes of globalization, Saskatchewan has assumed a pragmatic approach to federal-provincial relations. Most often, Saskatchewan has not been in favour of completely decentralizing policy-making. For instance, when the province initially proposed to develop the Saskatchewan Child Benefit, the province decided that it was not feasible or practical to implement this child benefit in isolation from other child welfare initiatives. The province spearheaded the concept of a National Child Benefit. Policies in Saskatchewan have usually been formulated after careful consideration of federal and provincial interests (Marchildon & Cotter, 2001).

Child-relevant policies in Canada and Saskatchewan are increasingly based on neo-liberal principles. For example, child poverty has been a policy priority of the federal and provincial governments since the notable House of Commons resolution in 1989. One of the main policy mechanisms introduced by the federal government to combat childhood poverty was the National Child Benefit (NCB). Yet, the NCB has entrenched and deepened the stigma attached to social assistance recipients. Since the Government of Saskatchewan does not provide the NCB to families on social assistance, Saskatchewan has created a clear distinction between the deserving and undeserving poor based on an attachment to the labour force (International Development Research Centre, n.d.; Wiegers, 2002). Furthermore, the Government of Saskatchewan's introduction of workfare represented the transfer of social responsibility from the state to the individual (Hunter & Miazdyck, 2003; International Development Research Centre, n.d.). Presenting the market and participation within this market as a panacea for social ills can be witnessed as a policy strategy across all of the Canadian provinces and territories (Hunter & Miazdyck, 2003; Hunter & Donovan, 2005).

CONCLUSION

Globalization, particularly since the 1980s, is synonymous with the neo-liberal policies that have been adopted by almost every government in the world (Teeple, 2000). Neo-liberalism has shaped the implementation of public policies in Canada, in Saskatchewan, and in Saskatoon that aim to privatize societal responsibility and/or delegate social responsibilities to other levels of governance, to communities, or to individuals. Child-relevant public policy of the federal, provincial, and sometimes municipal governments has been formulated according to a number of neo-liberal tenets. For instance, the primacy of the market is evident in a number of the child-relevant policies that were reviewed here. While these findings suggest that neo-liberalism has influenced Canadian and Saskatchewan child-relevant policy, there is some indication of a social investment strategy being pursued. Further analysis is required to determine the extent of a social investment strategy in Canada and Saskatchewan, although, in a number of ways, neo-liberalism and a social investment strategy are quite compatible. Both approaches to policy emphasize individualist, market-oriented solutions, although the latter promotes the importance of our youngest citizens for building a strong, prosperous society—or economy, which is often the more privileged marker of success under both approaches.

NOTES

1. The LICO is a standard used by Statistics Canada to compare wages and living expenses, where the value is the percentage of income that an average family spends on necessities including shelter, food, and clothing. A family falls below the LICO if the level of income is such that a typical family would spend more than 20 percent of that average income on necessities. This value is readjusted for community size and inflation.

REFERENCES

Baker, M. (1997). *The restructuring of the Canadian welfare state: Ideology and policy*. No. 77. Social Policy Research Centre.

Brown, D. M. (2002). Fiscal federalism: The new equilibrium between equity and efficiency. In H. Bakvis & G. Skogstad (Eds.), *Canadian federalism: Performance, effectiveness, and legitimacy* (pp. 59–84). Don Mills, ON: Oxford University Press.

Canadian Population Health Initiative. (2006). *Improving the health of Canadians: An introduction to health in urban places*. Ottawa: Canadian Institute for Health Information.

Carter, T., & Polevychok, C. (2004). *Housing is good social policy*. Ottawa: Canadian Policy Research Networks.

Childcare Resource and Research Unit. (1998). *Early childhood care and education in Canada: Provinces and territories*. Toronto: Childcare Resource and Research Unit, University of Toronto.

City of Saskatoon. (2006). *Housing business plan—2006—City of Saskatoon.* Saskatoon: City of Saskatoon.

Coburn, D. (2000). Income inequality, social cohesion and the health status of populations: The role of neo-liberalism. *Social Science Medicine, 51,* 135–146.

Coburn, D. (2004). Beyond the income inequality hypothesis: Class, neo-liberalism, and health inequalities. *Social Science Medicine, 58,* 41–56.

Cool, J. (2007). *Child care in Canada: The federal role.* No. 04–20E. Ottawa: Library of Parliament.

Cooper, M. (2001). *Housing affordability: A children's issue.* No. F|11. Ottawa: Canadian Policy Research Networks.

Cornia, G. A. (2001). Globalization and health: Results and options. *Bulletin of the World Health Organization, 79*(9), 834–841.

Cornia, G. A., & Kiiski, S. (2001). *Trends in income distribution in the post-World War II period: Evidence and interpretation.* Helsinki: UNU-WIDER.

Doherty, G., Friendly, M., & Beach, J. (2003). *OECD thematic review of early childhood education and care—Canadian background report.* Ottawa: Government of Canada.

Federal, Provincial and Territorial Ministers Responsible for Social Services. (2007). *The national child benefit progress report, 2005.* Ottawa: Government of Canada.

Foster, L., & Broad, D. (1998). *Summary report of flexible child care for flexible workers.* Regina: Social Policy Research Unit, University of Regina.

Fudge, J., & Cossman, B. (2002). Introduction: Privatization, law, and the challenge to feminism. In B. Cossman & J. Fudge (Eds.), *Privatization, law, and the challenge to feminism* (pp. 3–36). Toronto: University of Toronto Press.

Government of Canada. (1992). *Brighter futures: Canada's action plan for children.* Ottawa: Health and Welfare Canada.

Government of Canada. (1995). *A 21st century employment system for Canada: Guide to the employment insurance legislation.* Ottawa: Government of Canada.

Government of Canada. (2004). *A Canada fit for children: Canada's plan of action in response to the May 2002 United Nations special session on children.* Ottawa: Government of Canada.

Government of Saskatchewan. (n.d.). *Our children. Our promise. Our future. Early childhood development progress report 2004/2005.* Regina: Government of Saskatchewan.

Government of Saskatchewan. (1993). *Children First: An invitation to work together: Saskatchewan's action plan for children.* Regina: Interdepartmental Steering Committee.

Government of Saskatchewan. (1996). *Redesigning social assistance: Preparing for the new century.* Regina: Government of Saskatchewan.

Government of Saskatchewan. (1999). *Building on community success: Creating a long term plan for Saskatchewan's youngest children and their families.* Regina: Government of Saskatchewan.

Government of Saskatchewan. (2005). *2005 annual report—Saskatchewan housing corporation.* Regina: Government of Saskatchewan.

Government of Saskatchewan. (2008). *Minimum wage increase announced.* Accessed September 23, 2008, from http://www.gov.sk.ca/news?newsId=7fa94dc1-01b2-421b-af89-20f100aff108

Harvey, D. (2005). *A brief history of neoliberalism.* New York: Oxford University Press.

Hay, C. (2006). Globalization and public policy. In M. Moran, M. Rein, & R. E. Goodin (Eds.), *The Oxford handbook of public policy* (pp. 587–604). New York: Oxford University Press.

Hertzman, C. (2000). The case for an early childhood development strategy. *Canadian Journal of Policy Research, 1*(2), 11–18.

Hertzman, C. (May 2004). *Making early childhood development a priority: Lessons from Vancouver.* Vancouver, B.C.: Canadian Centre for Policy Alternatives.

Human Resources and Social Development Canada. (n.d.). *Social assistance statistical report: 2005.* Retrieved February 8, 2008, from http://www.hrsdc.gc.ca/

Hunter, G., & Donovan, K. (2005). *Transitional employment allowance, flat rate utilities, rental housing supplements and poverty in Saskatchewan.* Regina: Social Policy Research Unit, University of Regina.

Hunter, G., & Miazdyck, D. (2003). *Current issues surrounding poverty and welfare programming in Canada: Two reviews.* Regina: Social Policy Research Unit, University of Regina.

International Development Research Centre. (n.d.). *Formal income support provisions: Delineating and evaluating the impact of change.* Retrieved February 8, 2008, from http://archive.idrc.ca/socdev/pub/social/secta.html

Inwood, G. J. (2005). *Continentalizing Canada: The politics and legacy of the Macdonald Royal Commission.* Toronto: University of Toronto Press.

Irwin, L. G., Siddiqi, A., & Hertzman, C. (2007). *Early child development: A powerful equalizer.* World Health Organization.

Ismael, S. (2006). *Child poverty and the Canadian welfare state: From entitlement to charity.* Edmonton: University of Alberta Press.

Jenson, J., & Thompson, S. (1999). *Comparative family policy: Six provincial stories.* No. F|08. [Ottawa]: Canadian Policy Research Networks.

Kamerman, S. B., Neuman, M., Waldfogel, J., & Brooks-Gunn, J. (2003). *Social policies, family types, and child outcomes in selected OECD countries.* No. 6. Paris: Organisation for Economic Cooperation and Development.

Keating, D. P., & Mustard, J. F. (1993). Social economic factors and human development. In D. Ross (Ed.), *Family security in insecure times* (pp. 87–105). Ottawa: National Forum on Family Security.

Keil, R. (2002). "Common–Sense" neoliberalism: Progressive conservative urbanism in Toronto, Canada. *Antipode, 34*(3), 578–601.

Kindig, D., & Stoddart, G. (2003). What is population health? *American Journal of Public Health, 93*(3), 380–382.

Labonte, R., & Torgerson, R. (2005). Interrogating globalization, health and development: Towards a comprehensive framework for research, policy and political action. *Critical Public Health, 15*(2), 157–179.

Laurent, S., & Vaillancourt, F. (2004). *Federal-provincial transfers for social programs in Canada: Their status in May 2004.* No. 2004–07. Montreal: Institute for Research on Public Policy.

Lin, X. (1998). *Employment insurance in Canada: Recent trends and policy changes.* No. 125. Ottawa: Statistics Canada.

Low, M. D., Low, B. J., Baumler, E. R., & Huynh, P. T. (2005). Can education policy be health policy? Implications of research on the social determinants of health. *Journal of Politics, Policy and Law, 30*(6), 1131–1162.

Mahon, R. (2001). *School-aged children across Canada: A patchwork of public policies.* No. F|10. [Ottawa]: Canadian Policy Research Networks.

Maki, D., Friesen, J., & Siedule, T. (2001). *The influence of legislative changes to unemployment insurance on the economy 1971–94: A full-system simulation study (a non-technical summary).* Hull: Human Resources Development Canada.

Marchildon, G. P., & Cotter, B. (2001). Saskatchewan and the social union. In H. A. Leeson (Ed.), *Saskatchewan politics: Into the twenty-first century* (pp. 367–380). Regina, SK: Canadian Plains Research Center.

McBride, S. (2005). *Paradigm shift: Globalization and the Canadian state* (2nd ed.). Halifax, NS: Fernwood Publishing.

McIntosh, T., Muhajarine, N., & Klatt, B. (2004). *Understanding the policy landscape of early childhood development in Saskatchewan.* Saskatchewan Population Health and Evaluation Research Unit.

Merriman, T., & Pringle, B. (2008). *Affordable housing: An investment.* Regina: Task Force on Housing Affordability, Ministry of Social Services.

Muhajarine, N., Evitts, T., Horn, M., Glacken, J., & Pushor, D. (2007). *Full-time kindergarten in Saskatchewan, part two: An evaluation of full-time kindergarten programs in three school divisions.* Saskatoon: Community-University Institute for Social Research.

National Council of Welfare. (1995). *The 1995 budget and block funding.* Ottawa: Minister of Supply and Services Canada.

National Council of Welfare. (Spring 1997). *Child benefits: A small step forward.* National Council of Welfare.

National Council of Welfare. (Winter 2008). *Welfare incomes, 2006 and 2007.* Volume #128. Ottawa: National Council of Welfare.

Raphael, D. (2007). *Poverty and policy in Canada: Implications for health and quality of life.* Toronto: Canadian Scholars' Press, Inc.

Ruggeri, J. (2005). The evolution of provincial responsibility. In H. Lazar (Ed.), *Canadian fiscal arrangements: What works, what might work better* (pp. 83–126). Montreal: McGill-Queen's University Press.

Saint-Martin, D. (2007). From the welfare state to the social investment state: A new paradigm for Canadian social policy? In M. Orsini & M. Smith (Eds.), *Critical policy studies* (pp. 279–298). Vancouver: UBC Press.

Sancton, A. (2002). Municipalities, cities, and globalization: Implications for Canadian federalism. In H. Bakvis & G. Skogstad (Eds.), *Canadian federalism: Performance, effectiveness, and legitimacy* (pp. 261–277). Don Mills, ON: Oxford University Press.

Saskatchewan Minimum Wage Board. (2007). *Report to the Minister of Labour on the minimum wage and other matters under section 15 of the Labour Standards Act.* Regina: Saskatchewan Minimum Wage Board.

Saunders, R. (2005). *Low-paid workers in Saskatchewan.* Ottawa: Canadian Policy Research Networks.

Smith, N. (2002). New globalism, new urbanism: Gentrification as global urban strategy. *Antipode, 34*(3), 427–450.

Stren, R., & Polese, M. (2000). Understanding the new sociocultural dynamics of cities: Comparative urban policy in global context. In R. Stren & M. Polese (Eds.), *The social sustainability of cities: Diversity and the management of change* (pp. 3–38). Toronto: University of Toronto Press.

Tanzi, V. (2006). Making policy under efficiency pressures: Globalization, public spending, and social welfare. In I. Kaul & P. Conceicao (Eds.), *The new public finance: Responding to global challenges* (pp. 109–130). New York: Oxford University Press.

Teeple, G. (2000). *Globalization and the decline of social reform: Into the twenty-first century.* Aurora: Garamond Press.

Thompson, R. (2002). Developmental-ecological considerations. In N. H. Kaufman & I. Rizzini (Eds.), *Globalization and children: Exploring potentials for enhancing opportunities in the lives of children and youth* (pp. 107–114). New York, NY: Kluwer Academic/Plenum Publishers.

Wade, R. H. (2004). Is globalization reducing poverty and inequality? *International Journal of Health Services, 34*(3), 318–414.

Wallerstein, N. (1992). Powerlessness, empowerment, and health: Implications for health promotion programs. *American Journal of Health Promotion, 6*(3), 197–205.

Warnock, J. W. (2003). *The structural adjustment of capitalism in Saskatchewan.* Saskatoon, SK: Canadian Centre for Policy Alternatives.

White, L. A. (2002). The child care agenda and the social union. In H. Bakvis & G. Skogstad (Eds.), *Canadian federalism: Performance, effectiveness, and legitimacy* (pp. 105–123). Don Mills, ON: Oxford University Press.

Wiegers, W. (2002). *The framing of poverty as "child poverty" and its implications for women.* [Ottawa]: Status of Women Canada.

Wilkinson, R. (1992). Income distribution and life expectancy. *British Medical Journal, 304,* 165–168.

Young, T. K. (2004). *Population health: Concepts and methods* (2nd ed.). New York: Oxford University Press.

List of Contributors

SYLVIA ABONYI is an Associate Professor in the Department of Community Health and Epidemiology at the University of Saskatchewan, Research Faculty with the Saskatchewan Population Health and Evaluation Research Unit, and a Canada Research Chair in Aboriginal Health

ANGELA BOWEN is an Associate Professor at the College of Nursing, an Associate Member of the Department of Psychiatry, College of Medicine, University of Saskatchewan, and a Community Population Health Research training program alumnus.

KELLY CHESSIE is a PhD candidate in Interdisciplinary Studies at the University of Saskatchewan and a Community Population Health Research training program alumnus.

JENNIFER CUSHON is a PhD candidate in Community Health and Epidemiology at the University of Saskatchewan.

J. DAVID GUERRERO is a PhD candidate with the Department of Philosophy at the University of Calgary.

JANELLE HIPPE is a Community Population Health Research training program alumnus and a PhD student in sociology at Queen's University in Kingston.

BONNIE JEFFERY is a Professor of Social Work and Director of the Saskatchewan Population Health and Evaluation Research Unit at the University of Regina.

SHANTHI JOHNSON is a Professor and Associate Dean (Research and Graduate Studies) with the Faculty of Kinesiology and Health Studies and Research Faculty with the Saskatchewan Population health and Evaluation Research Unit at the University of Regina.

TOM MCINTOSH is an Associate Professor of Political Science and Research Faculty with the Saskatchewan Population Health and Evaluation Research Unit at the University of Regina.

DIANE MARTZ is the Director with the Research Ethics Office and Research Faculty with the Saskatchewan Population Health and Evaluation Research Unit at the University of Saskatchewan.

NAZEEM MUHAJARINE is a Professor of Community Health and Epidemiology and Research Faculty at Saskatchewan Population Health and Evaluation Research Unit at the University of Saskatchewan.

NADINE NOWATZKI is a PhD candidate in the Department of Sociology at the University of Manitoba.

ANDRÉ PICARD is the national health reporter for the *Globe and Mail*.

RHONA SHAW is a Post-Doctoral Fellow in the Department of Sociology at the University of Saskatchewan.

ULRICH TEUCHER is an Assistant Professor in the Program of Culture and Human Development, Department of Psychology, and Co-director of the Qualitative Research Centre at the University of Saskatchewan.

index

A

Abel, T., 45, 49

Abelson, J., 76–77, 87, 89

Abonyi, S., xvi, xxi, xxv, 30, 32–34

Aboriginal communities, 16, 29, 42, 60, 65, 136; cultural differences among, 58, 62, 70; knowledge systems of, 58, 63–64, 66, 70; language families of, 62; and population health, xiii, xxii, 27; self-government and suicide rates, 68–69

Aboriginal identity: and pregnancy care, 94, 96, 101, 103–5, 107, 109, 136

Aboriginal youth: suicide rates of, xxii, 57–58, 67–70

Achieving health for all: A framework for health promotion, 90

Action Plan for Children (SK), 155

Adams, D., 78, 89, 92

Adler, P., 118, 130

Adler, P.A., 118, 130

Affordable housing: An investment, 167

Agendas, alternatives and public policies, xxv

Ainsworth, B., 119, 132

Alexandra, H., 148

Almeder, R.F., 18

Alspac Study Team, The, 149

Amaratunga, C., 89

Amaro, H., 150

America in 1492: The world of the Indian peoples before the arrival of Columbus, 72

American Indian mind in a linear world: American Indian studies and traditional knowledge, The, 71

American Indian thought: Philosophical essays, 71, 73

American Psychiatric Association, 134, 148

Analyzing social settings: A guide to qualitative observation and analysis, 110

Anderson, B., 125, 130

Anderson, M., xvi, xxv

Arcury, T.A., 96, 109

Ariew, A., 18

Aristotle, 14, 17–18

Arman, M., 127, 130

Armstrong, D., 96, 109

Armstrong, H., 42, 49

Armstrong, P., 42, 49, 86, 89

Arnstein, S.R., 77, 87, 89

B

Baetz, M., 148

Baggott, R., 77, 89

Baker, John A., 17

Baker, M., 156, 164

Bakvis, H., 164, 167–68

Balfour, J., 50–51

Ball, J., 30, 32, 67

Ball, L., 71

Barer, M.L., 52

Barker, D.J.P., 135, 147–48

Barker, K.K., 93, 109

Barnes, J., 18

Barnett, E., 77, 90

Barry, K.L., 149

Battiste, M., 59, 61–64, 66, 71

Bauchner, H., 150

Baum, F.E., 53

Baumler, E.R., 166

Beach, J., 159, 165

Beck, U., 95, 109

Beckfield, J., 37, 49

Belmont report: Ethical principles and guidelines for the protection of human subjects of research, The, 27, 32–33

Benach, J., 52

Bennett, H., 148

Benzeval, M., 37, 50

Berkman, L., 50–51

Bernard, C., 149

Bernier, J., 89

Bierwert, Crisca, 64, 71

Bill C-12, 161

Bindon, J.R., xvi, xxv

biostatistical theory (BST), 10–13

Blake, J.S., 62, 72

Blalock, H.M., 22–26, 32

Blanchard, C., 116, 130

Blanchard, J., 30, 33

Blazer, D.G., 134, 136, 142, 148

Blinde, E., 123, 130

Blow, F.C., 149

Bobak, M., 41, 51–52

Boctor, M.A., 109

Bogdon, R., 118, 130

Bolla, P., 128, 131

Bonari, L., 135, 148

Bond, A., 150

Boorse, Christopher, 10–11, 17–18

Borrell, C., 52

Bosma, H., 71

Bourdieu, Pierre, 44–46, 109

Bowen, Angela, xxiii, 135, 137, 144, 147–48

Bowring, F., 45, 49

Bramley, D., xvi, xxv

Brawley, L., 116, 130

Breakwell, G., 118, 130

breast cancer, x, 117, 121, 129; diagnosis of, 127–28; and dragon boating, 116, 118, 126; supportive care for, xxiii, 115, 123–24; treatment for, 115, 119, 122, 125, 127–28. *See also* dragon boat racing

Bredin, M., 125, 130

Brief history of neoliberalism, A., 165

Brighter futures: Canada's action plan for children, 155, 165

British Columbia Centre of Excellence for Women's Health, 107

British Columbia, University of, 71

Broad, D., 158–59, 165

Broadhead, E., 116, 130

Brody, H., 64–65, 71

Brooks-Gunn, J., 166

Brown, Annette, 94, 107, 109

Brown, D.M., 153, 164

Brueckner, I., xxv

Brushed by cedar, living by the river: Coast Salish figures of power, 71

Building Independence— Investing in Families, 157

Building on community success: Creating a long term plan for Saskatchewan's youngest children and their families, 165

Building on values: The future of health care in Canada— final report, xxv

Burchill, C.A., xvi, xxv

Burstrom, B., 53

Bynum, W.F., 18

C

Cabral, H., 150

Cain, C., 61, 72

Calnan, M., 95, 111

Calvert, Lorne, 79, 83

Cammer, A., 33

Campbell, J.C., 94, 109

Canada fit for children: Canada's plan of action in response to the May 2002 United Nations special session on children, A, 165

Canada, Government of, 158, 161, 165

Canada Health and Social Transfer (CHST), 157

Canada Health Transfer (CHT), 157

Canada Social Transfer (CST), 157

Canadian Assistance Plan (CAP), 161; elimination of, 157, 162

Canadian Cancer Society, 115, 130

Canadian Community Health Survey, 24, 30, 32

Canadian fact book on poverty 1994, 111

Canadian federalism: Performance, effectiveness, and legitimacy, 164, 167–68

Canadian fiscal arrangements: What works, what might work better, 167

Canadian Institute for Health Information (CIHI), 32

Canadian Institutes of Health Research (CIHR), xi, 27, 30, 32, 71, 146–47

Canadian Policy Research Networks, 155

Canadian Population Health Initiative, 154, 164

Canadian Public Health Association (CPHA), 15, 18

Canadian Public Health Association response to the World Health Organization (WHO) Commission's report, 18

Canadian Research Index, 155

Canadian Social Research Links, 155

Cancer journals, The, 131

Canguilem, Georges, 20, 32

Caplan, Arthur, 9, 18–19, 135

Caplan, H.L., 148

Captured womb: A history of the medical care of pregnant women, The, 110

Caring for medicare: Sustaining a quality system, 90

Carpiano, R.M., 22, 24, 29, 32, 45, 48–49

Carter, T., 160, 164

Certain, L., 135, 149

Chandler, Michael J., 57–58, 67–69, 71

Change in nutrition and food security in two Inuit communities, 1992–1997, 33

Changing health care in Canada: The Romanow papers, 90

Charles, C., 77, 87, 89

Chassin, M., xxv

Cheers, B., 77, 92

Chessie, Kelly, xxii, 75–76, 86, 89–90

Child benefits: A small step forward, 167

child care agreements, bilateral, 158

Child care in Canada: The federal role, 165

child care program, ix, 154, 158–59. *See also* social programs

child health, xv, xvi, 155, 157; determinants for, 154; and dismantling of welfare state, 153; and globalization, xxiv, 154; and low-incomes, 152. *See also* fetal health; health determinants; infants

Child poverty and the Canadian welfare state: From entitlement to charity, 166

child-relevant public policy, xxiv, 154, 164

child welfare. *See* child health

Childcare Resource and Research Unit, 159, 164

Children First: An invitation to work together: Saskatchewan's action plan for children, 165

Chiu, H.F.K., 148

Choi, I., 59, 72

Choice in Child Care Allowance, 159

Chomik, T.A., 19

Christensen, R., 16, 18

Chung, T.K.H., 135, 142, 148

Church, J., 77, 89

Churchill, L.R., xxv

CIHR guidelines for health research involving Aboriginal peoples, 30, 32

Citizens: An underused and undervalued asset in the pursuit of improved health care delivery, 91

Citizens at the centre: Deliberative participation in health care decisions, 90

Clair, M., 75, 90

Clancy, C.M., xxv

Closer to home: Report of the British Columbia Royal Commission on health care and costs, 92

Closson, T., 75, 90

Coburn, D., 36, 42–43, 49, 153–54, 165

Cogill, S.R., 148

Cohen, R., 50–51

Cohen, S., 115, 131

Colburn, D., 49

Cole, B., 134, 148

Coleman, D., 116, 130

Coleman, J., 39, 49

College of Nursing (SK), 147

Collins, H.M., 77, 87, 90

Colman, R., 52

Colyer, H., 127, 130

Commission on the Future of Health Care, 89

Community Advisory Network (CAN), 79, 84–86

Community and Population Health Research (CPHR), xix-xx; Strategic Training Program, xi-xii, xviii, xx, 147; transdisciplinary scholarship of, xviii-xix

Community Child Care Investment Program, 159

Community participation in health-system decision making, 90

Community-University Institutes of Social Research (CUISR), 147

Companion encyclopedia of the history of medicine, 18

Comparative family policy: Six provincial stories, 166

Complete works of Aristotle: The revised Oxford translation, The, 18

Comprehensive textbook of psychiatry, 148

Conceicao, P., 167

Concepts of health and disease: Interdisciplinary perspectives, 19

Consequences of modernity, The, 110

Conservative Party (SK), 78, 89

Considerations for the development of public health surveillance in First Nations communities, 33

Constitution of the World Health Organization, 19

Continentalizing Canada: The politics and legacy of the Macdonald Royal Commission, 166

Cool, J., 158–59, 165

Cooper, M., 160, 165

Cooper, P.J., 135, 148–49

Cooper, R., 17–18

Coping and self-concept in adolescence, 71

Corin, E., 22, 33

Cornelius, M.D., 149

Cornia, G.A., 154, 165

Cossman, B., 152–53, 165

Cotter, B., 163, 167

Counterrevolution and revolt, 72

Courneya, K., 116, 130

Coustan, D., 150

Cox, J.L., 138, 148–49

Crichton, A., 74, 90

Critical policy studies, 167

Crouch, M., 124–25, 131

Crowther, C.A., 136, 150

Culos-Reed, N., 116, 130

culture: as health determinant, xvi, 68–69

Culture power place: Explorations in critical anthropology, 72

Culture's consequences: International differences in work-related values, 72

Cunningham, C., 59, 71

Current issues surrounding poverty and welfare programming in Canada: Two reviews, 166

Cushon, Jennifer, xxiv

Custer died for your sins—an Indian manifesto, 71

Cyranowski, J., 125, 130

D

Daiuth, C., 71

Dakota people: A history of the Dakota, Lakota and Nakota through 1863, 72

Daley, D.M., 22, 24, 29, 32, 48–49

Daniels, N., 35, 49

Danis, M., xxv

D'Arcy, C., 94, 110

Das Mittelalter: Geschichte und Kultur, 71

Dattilo, J., 131

Davey Smith, G., 39–40, 43, 47–52

Davidson, N., 35, 53

Davies, C., 77, 90

Davis, C., 130

Davis, M.S., 90–91

Dawson, D., 128, 131

Day, N.L., 149

Dean, R.S., 150

Deaton, A., 37, 49

Deber, R.B., 74, 76, 90–91

Declaration of Helsinki, 27, 32, 34

Deem, R., 119, 130

Delaquis, S., 75, 90

DeLong-Gierveld, J.J., 32

Deloria, V., 61–62, 71

DeMaio, S., 77, 87, 89

Demos, V., 53

Denzin, N., 130

depression, viii, xxiii, 145; effects of, 133, 135–36, 142, 146; and health determinants, xxiii, 135–36; as population health problem, 134; in postpartum women, 135–36, 138; during pregnancy, 133–35, 141, 144, 146; prevention of, 133, 139–40, 144, 146–47; screening for, 142–44, 146; treatment for, 136, 138–39, 142–43, 146. *See also* fetal health

DesMeules, M, xvi, xxv

Developing a healthy communities index: A collection of papers, 33

Development as freedom, 52

Devine, Grant, 89

diabetes, gestational, 135

Dickinson, H.D., 77, 90–91

Diderichsen, F., 53

Dim, J., 149

Disability Adjusted Life Years (DALYS), 134

Discipline and punish, 110

disease prevention, viii, xxii, 74, 80, 139, 142

Distinction: A social critique of the judgment of taste, 109

Doctors of infamy: The story of the Nazi medical crimes, 33

Doherty, G., 159, 165

Donovan, K., 158, 163, 166

Dorgan, M., 89

Dorland, J., 90–91

Douglas, T.C., 78, 80

Dr. Susan Love's breast book, 131

Drache, D., 74, 90–91

dragon boat racing: experiences of, xxiii, 116–18, 122, 129; as physical activity, 119, 123; team as support group, 115, 120–28

Dressler, W.W., xvi, xxv

Due, P., 51

Duleep, H.O., 36, 50

DuMont, J., 110

Duncan, K., xvi, xxv, 33

Dunkel-Schetter, C., 110

Dunn, J.R., 52

Duran, B., 61, 71

Duran, E., 61, 71

Durkheim, E., 35, 40, 50

Dutchak, J.J., 91

Dwellings: A spiritual history of the living world, 72

Dwyer, J., 76, 90

Dyck, R., 94, 109

E

Early child development: A powerful equalizer, 166

Early childhood care and education in Canada: Provinces and territories, 164

early childhood development, 156, 159, 162. *See also* child health

Early Childhood Development initiative, 156

early childhood policy, 154

Edinburgh Postnatal Depression Scale (EPDS), 138

education: as health determinant, 11, 35, 42

Einerson, A., 148

Ellaway, A., 38, 50

Elvin, N., 115–16, 132

Emerging solutions: Report and recommendations, 90

emotional support: for cancer survivors, 122

Employment Insurance (EI), 155, 161; and restructuring UI/EI system, 161–62

Employment insurance in Canada: Recent trends and policy changes, 166

Endicott, J., 136, 149

Engelhardt Jr, H.T., 19

Epidemiology, 148

Epp, J., 88, 90

Ereshefsky, M., 17, 19

Ermine, W.J., xxi, 21–22, 30, 33

Established Programs Financing (EPF), 157

Estabrooks, C.A., 91

Ethical dimensions of health policy, xxv

ethics: in population health research, 21–22

Ethics: Inventing right and wrong, 19

Ethics and the metaphysics of medicine, 19

Evaluation frameworks for the Aboriginal health human resources initiative and the Aboriginal health transition fund, 34

Evans, J., 148

Evans, R.G., 52, 77, 87, 90

Evitts, T., 167

Exposing privatization: Women and health care reform in Canada, 89

Eyels, J., 89

F

Fairclough, N., 77, 90

Family Health Benefit (FHB), 157

Family security in insecure times, 166

Farrant, W., 90

Fasting, K., 128, 130

Fat, D., 149

Feather, J., 89–90

Federal, Provincial and Territorial Ministers Responsible for Social Services, 156, 165

Federal-provincial transfers for social programs in Canada: Their status in May 2004, 166

Federalism, democracy and health policy in Canada, 92

"Feelings in Pregnancy and Motherhood Study," 134, 136, 138, 147

Feldman, P.J., 94, 110

Ferguson, J., 65, 72

fetal health: and maternal depression, 146; negative effects on, 136, 142; promotion of, 144, 147; well-being of, 140, 146. *See also* depression; infants

Field, T., 135, 148

Fife-Shaw, C., 130

First Nations communities. *See* Aboriginal communities

First Nations, Inuit, and Aboriginal health, 72

Fiske, Jo-Anne, 107, 109

Fitch, M., 130

Fixico, D.F., 59, 71

Flynn, H.A., 149

Forest, P.G., 89–90

Formal income support provisions: Delineating and evaluating the impact of change, 166

Foster, L., 158–59, 165

Foucault, Michael, 94–96, 98, 106, 110

Foundations of social theory, The, 49

Framework for reform: Report of the Premier's Advisory Council on Health, A, 91

Framing of poverty as "child poverty" and its implications for women, 168

Frankish, C.J., 6–7, 17, 19, 75, 90

Fransoo, R., 30, 33

Fried, J., 60, 71

Friendly, M., 159, 165

Friesen, J., 161, 166

Fritzell, J., 53

Frohlich, K., 22, 33

Fudge, J., 152–53, 165

Fulford, K.W.M., 13, 19

Full-time kindergarten in Saskatchewan, part two: An evaluation of full-time kindergarten programs in three school divisions, 167

Functions: New essays in the philosophy of psychology and biology, 18

Future directions for health care in Saskatchewan, 92

Fyke Commission, 78–79

Fyke in the road: Health reform in Saskatchewan from Romanow to Calvert and beyond, The, 91

Fyke, K., 75, 83, 90

G

Galabuzi, G.E., 44, 50

Gandhi, L., 61, 72

Gatrell, A., 45, 50

Gauvin, F.P., 89

Gehlbach, S., 130

Gender inequality: Feminist theories and politics, 131

Gender perspectives in health and medicine: Key themes, 53

Gender, race, class and health: Intersectional approaches, 52

Geography of thought: How Asians and Westerns think differently ... and why, The, 59, 72

Gerdtham, U.G., 50

Giddens, Anthony, 94–95, 98, 110, 162

Gill, D., 128, 131

Gillham, L., 115, 130

Girl and the game. A history of women's sport in Canada, The, 130

Giving birth in Canada, 1900–1950, 110

Glacken, J., 33, 167

Glannon, Walter, 18

Global inequality and human needs: Health and illness in an increasingly unequal world, 53

globalization, xxiv, 151–52, 154, 163–64. *See also* welfare state

Globalization and children: Exploring potentials for enhancing opportunities in the lives of children and youth, 168

Globalization and the decline of social reform: Into the twenty-first century, 167

Globe and Mail, The, 73

Glover, T., 116, 130

Glover, V., 135, 148–49

Golding, J., 148

Goldschmidt, L., 149

Goodin, R.E., 165

Goodman, J.H., 136, 148

Goodyer, I.M., 149

Gordis, L., 142–43, 148

Gordon, C., 90

Goulet, L., 110

Grant, K., 89

Grant, L., 62, 72

Gravlee, C.C., xvi, xxv

Gray, J., 75, 90

Gray, R., 119, 130

Green, K., 33

Green, L.W., 19

Grimson, R., 130

Guerrero, J. David, xxi

Gupta, A., 65, 72

H

Habermas, J., 61, 72

Hackett, P., xxv, 33

Hall, L., 77, 92

Hall, M.A., 128, 130

Hallett, D., 57, 67–69, 71

Hammond, S., 130

Hampton, M., xxv, 33

Han, L., 123, 130

Handbook of bioethics, The, 19

Handbook of psychiatric measures, 148

Handbook of qualitative research, 130

Hankivsky, O., 46–47, 50

Hansen, P., 76, 90

Harper, S., 50

Harrington, M., 128, 131

Harris, S., 115–16, 131

Harvey, D., 20, 33, 151, 165

Hay, C., 153, 155, 165

Hayward, K., 52

Healing traditions: The mental health of Aboriginal peoples in Canada, 71

health: as correlated with income, viii, xiii, xxi, 37, 47–48; definition of, 3–4, 8–10, 15; determinants of, vii-viii, 4, 11, 21, 35, 49, 116; minimum standard of, 7–8, 11–12, 15–16; promotion of, xxii, 74, 80; and values, 9–14. *See also* child health; health determinants; population health

health advice phone line, 83

Health and social change: A critical theory, 52

Health Canada, 4, 8, 16–17, 19, 57, 72, 155

Health care: A community concern?, 90

Health care ethics: An introduction, 18

health care policy, 87–88

health care system, ix-x, 15, 42, 89, 128; community involvement in, 74, 76, 80–81, 85, 87, 89; governance for, 75, 77, 82, 88; outcomes of, 35, 43, 47

health determinants, xvi, xxii, 14, 22, 47, 140–41, 144, 152, 154; of depression, 135–36, 139, 146–47

health disparities, 11–12, 36, 38, 41, 43–44, 47, 139, 143; and population health research, 14, 20; reduction of, xiv, xxi, 9, 15–16, 21, 58, 69. *See also* income distribution; social differences

health facility boards, 75, 81, 84, 86

Health Impact Assessment (HIA), 150

Health impact assessment as a tool for population health promotion and public policy, 19

health inequalities. *See* health disparities

Health insurance and Canadian public policy: The seven decisions that created the Canadian Health Insurance System, 92

Health of nations: Why inequality is harmful to your health, 50

health promotion. *See* health, promotion of

Health systems in transition: Canada, 91

Healthier societies: From analysis to action, 52

Healthy Mother Healthy Baby Program, 136–38, 144, 146–47

Healthy people, a healthy province: the action plan for Saskatchewan health care, 83, 92

Heidegger, M., 63, 72

Helgeson, V., 115, 131

Hellin, D., 135, 148

Heraclitus, 63

Herbert, P., xxv

Heron, J., 136, 142, 148–49

Hertzman, C., 52, 154, 166

Heyden, S., 130

Heymann, J., 52

Hidden actors, muted voices: The employment of rural women in Saskatchewan forestry and agri-food industries, xxv

Hillemeier, M., 50–51

Himes, M., 125, 131

Hippe, Janelle, xxiii

Hipwell, A., 135, 149

Hiscock, R., 50

History of sexuality, The, 110

Hofstede, G., 59, 72

Hogan, L., 60, 72

Holden, J.M., 138, 148

Holland, D., 61, 72

Horn, M., 167

House, J., 51

House of Commons resolution (1989): on child poverty, 163

Housing affordability: A children's issue, 165

Housing Business Plan, 160

Housing business plan— 2006—City of Saskatoon, 165

Housing is good social policy, 164

housing policy, 154, 159–60. *See also* social housing

Houston, C.S., 89–90

How healthy are rural Canadians? An assessment of their health status and health determinants, xvi, xxv

How many roads? Regionalization and decentralization in health care, 90–91

Hox, J., 32

Huberman, M.A., 98, 110

Hugi, M., 131

Human Resources and Social Development Canada, 157, 166

Humber, J.M., 18

Hunter, G., 157–58, 163, 166

Hunters and bureaucrats: Power, knowledge, and aboriginal-state relations in the southwest Yukon, 72

Hurley, J., 91

Hutchinson, S., 116–17, 131

Huynh, P.T., 166

Hyndman, L., 74, 77, 90

I

Identity and agency in cultural worlds, 72

Impact of inequality: How to make sick societies healthier, The, 53

Improving the health of Canadians: An introduction to health urban places, 164

Inclusive society, The? Social exclusion and new labour, 50

income, vii, x; as health determinant, viii, xxi, 15, 35

income distribution, ix, 41, 49; inequalities in, xxii, 36–37, 42–43, 47–48, 154; and population health research, xxi. *See also* health disparities

income inequality hypothesis, 36–37, 48

Indigenous communities. *See* Aboriginal communities

Indigenous cultures in an interconnected world, 73

Individualism and collectivism, 73

Inequalities in health: The Black report, 53

Inequality is bad for our hearts: Why low income and social exclusion are major causes of heart disease in Canada, 52

infants: health determinants for, 135, 154. *See also* fetal health

Influence of legislative changes to unemployment insurance on the economy 1971–94, The, 166

Inhorn, M.C., 46–47, 53

Inoue, M., 149

Interagency Advisory Panel on Research Ethics, 28–29, 33

International Development Research Centre, 158, 163, 166

Intimate enemy: Loss and recovery of self under colonialism, The, 72

Introduction to critical discourse analysis in education, An, 92

Introduction to qualitative research methods: A phenomenological approach to the social sciences, 130

Inwood, G.J., 152, 166

Ireson, C., 77, 92

Irwin, L.G., 154, 166

Is inequality bad for our health?, 49

Islam, M.K., 39–40, 50

Ismael, S., 161–62, 166

Iso-Ahola, S., 116, 130–31

Iwasaki, Y., 116, 131

J

Jacklin, K., 30, 33

Jackson, S., 71

Jacobs Kronenfeld, J., 53

James, K., 59, 72

James, S., 130

Janyst, P., 30, 32

Jebamani, L.S., xvi, xxv

Jeffery, B., xvi, xxv, 22, 30–34

Jenson, J., 155, 157, 159, 161, 166

Jespersen, D., 116, 131

Joffres, M.R., 94, 111

Johnson, S., xxv, 21, 28–31, 33–34

Johnston, xx, xiv

Jokelainen, J., 149

Josephy, Jr., a.m., 72

Joukamaa, M., 149

Judge, K., 37, 50

Jumper Thurman, P., 33

K

Kahn, R.S., 135, 149

Kamerman, S.B., 159, 161, 166

Kane, C., 148

Kaplan, B., 130

Kaplan, G.A., 35, 38, 40–41, 43, 47–48, 50–52

Kass, L., 5, 19

Katula, J., 128, 131

Katz, R., 148

Kaufman, N.H., 168

Kaul, I., 167

Kawachi, I., 35, 37–40, 48–51, 53

Kearns, A., 50

Keating, D.P., 154, 166

Keefe, J., 77, 86, 92

Keil, R., 151, 166

Kennedy, B.P., 35, 38–39, 48–50

Khushf, G., 17, 19

KidsFirst Program, 157; evaluation Phase 1, 33

Kidwell, C.S., 61, 72

Kiiski, S., 154, 165

Killeen, M., 148

Kindig, D., 139, 149, 155, 166

Kingdon, J.W., xiii, xxv

Kinoshameg, P., 30, 33

Kirmayer, L., 34, 57, 71–72

Kitayama, S., 59, 72

Klatt, B., 161, 167

Klebaum, N., 148

Kleiber, D., 116, 131

Klomp, H., 109

knowledge, 59–60, 64;
transfer of, xvii, xxiv,
58, 61–63, 66, 69–70
knowledge, expert, 95, 97–
101, 105; and agency of
pregnant women, 93, 106
knowledge, Indigenous, 58–
64, 66, 69, 71
knowledge, Western, 64, 69
Koch, T., 24, 33
Koren, G., 148
Kostaras, X., 149
Kouri, D., 75–76, 90–91
Kramer, M.S., 94, 110
Kraus, P., 125, 131
Krell, D.F., 72
Kubzansky, L.D., 40, 50
Kumar, R., 148
Kurlowicz, L., 148
Kwan, B., 90

L

Labonte, R., xii-xiii, xvi, xxv,
33, 39, 43–44, 50, 52,
151, 166
labour policy, 154, 161
*Labour relations and health
reform: A comparative
study of five jurisdictions,*
92
Laing, D., 116, 130
Lalonde, c.e., 31, 33, 57–58,
67–69, 71
Lalonde report, 15
Lancet, The, xiv
Lane, K., 116, 131
Language and power, 90
Lanichotte, W., 61, 72
Larsen, C., 19
Lau, K., 148
Laurent, S., 156, 158, 166
Lawn, J., 20, 33
Lazar, H., 167
Lazarus, Ellen, 106, 110
Le normal et le pathologique, 20
Leader, A., 94, 110
Lee, D.T.S., 148

Leeson, H.A., 89, 167
Legislative Assembly of
Saskatchewan, 78, 90–91
LeMaster, P.L., 33
Leppin, A., 116, 132
Levine, M., 131
Levitas, R., 45, 50
Lewis, S., 75–76, 86, 90–91
Liberal Party (Fed), 158
Liberal Party (SK), 78
Liepert, R., 75, 91
Lightfoot, C., 71
Limits of medicine, The, 19
Lin, X., 160–61, 166
Lincoln, Y., 130
Lindstrom, M., 50
Link, B., 50
Little Bear, L., 66, 72
*Local Health System
Integration Act, 2006,* 90
Lochner, K., 50
Lockhead, C., 109, 111
Lofland, J., 98, 110
Lofland, L.H., 98, 110
Lomas, J., 75, 77, 86, 91–92
Lorber, J., 117, 131
Lorde, A., 125, 131
Love, S., 128, 131
Low, B.J., 166
Low-Income Cut-Off
(LICO), 161, 164
Low, M.D., 155, 166
*Low-paid workers in
Saskatchewan,* 167
Loy, D., 131
Lubotsky, D., 37, 49
Lundber, O., 53
Luo, Z.-C., 94, 110
Lydon, J., 110
Lynch, J.W., 35, 37–43,
47–52

M

Macdonald Commission, 152
MacDonald, J., 52
MacDougall, C., 53

Macinko, J.A., 37–38, 40,
48, 51
Macintyre, S., 50
Mackie, J.L., 17, 19
MacKinnon, M.P., 77, 91
Macleod, J., 39–40, 51
Mahon, R., 156, 162–63, 166
Maki, D., 161, 166
Maki, P., 135, 149
*Making democracy work:
Civic traditions in
modern Italy,* 52
*Making early childhood devel-
opment a priority: Lessons
from Vancouver,* 166
Mannell, R., 116, 131
*Maps and dreams: Indians
and the British Columbia
frontier,* 71
Marchildon, G.P., 76, 78–79,
90–91, 163, 167
Marcus, S.M., 134, 149
Marcuse, H., 65, 72
*Market limits in health reform:
Public success, private
failure,* 90–91
Markus, H.R., 59, 72
Marmot, Michael, viii, 35, 41,
44, 47, 51–53
Martens, P.J., xvi, xxv, 30, 33
Martin, E., 89
*Martin Heidegger: Basic writ-
ings,* 72
Martz, D., xvii, xxv, 33–34
Marx, Karl, 40, 42
Massie, M., 127, 131
Maternal Mental Health
Advisory Committee, 144
Maternal Mental Health Pro-
gram, 144, 147
Mathers, C.D., 134, 149
Mazankowski, D., 75, 91
McBride, S., 151, 153,
157, 167
McCall, L., 46, 51
McCallum, A., 77, 87, 92
McCartney, J.J., 19
McDermott, R., 94, 110

McDowell, L., 65, 72

McGarvey, S., 150

Mcintosh, M., xxv

McIntosh, T., xxv, 33–34, 78–79, 90–91, 161, 167

McKay, L., 50

McKee, N., 148

McKenzie, D., 116, 131

McKenzie, H., 124–25, 131

medicare, ix, 75, 79, 83

Mellor, J.M., 37, 51

Mental Health Evidence and Research (MER), 150

mental health, maternal, 140, 146; and depression, 133. *See also* depression; pregnancy

Mental health of Canadian Aboriginal peoples: Transformations of identity and community, 34

Merlo, J., 50

Merriman, T., 160, 167

Methods of critical discourse analysis, 92

Métis communities, 136

Meyer, M., 77, 92

Mhatre, S.L., 74, 91

Miazdyck, D., 157–58, 163, 166

Michael Smith Foundation (MSFHR), 71

Microlog, 155

Mielke, F., 32–33

Miles, M.B., 98, 110

Miller, P., 96, 111

Mills, S., xxv

Milyo, J., 37, 51

minimum wage, ix, 161

Minimum wage increase announced, 165

Ministry of Health annual report 2005-2006, 92

Ministry of Health, SK, 79

Misri, S., 136, 149

Mitchell, T., 116, 131

Mitchinson, W., 93, 110

Mitscherlich, A., 32–33

Miyo-Mahcihowin: A report on Indigenous health in Saskatchewan, xxv

Mo-Tzu, 63

Moesgaard-Iburg, K., 149

Mohr, W., 148

Moral Theory and Medical Practice, 19

Moran, M., 165

Mordacci, R., 5, 19

Morgan, K.P., 94, 110

Morgan, L., 77, 91

Morimoto, K., 149

Moving population and public health knowledge into action, 32

Muhajarine, Nazeem, xxiii–xxv, 30, 33, 94, 110, 135, 147–48, 159, 161, 167

Mulligan, J., 37, 50

Mullings, L., 46, 52

Mulroney, Brian, 158

Multilateral Framework Agreement on Early Learning and Child Care, 158

Muntaner, C., 37, 39, 42, 47–48, 51–52

Muramaki, J., 139, 149

Murphy, C.C., 94, 110

Murray Commission, 78, 89

Murray, D., 138, 149

Murray, L., 135, 148–9

Murray, R.G., 74, 77, 92

Mustard, C., 91, 154

Mustard, J.F., 166

Mustin, K., 128, 131

Myhr, T.I., 110

N

Nadasdy, P., 59, 72

Nandy, A., 61, 72

Narrative analysis: Studying the development of individuals in society, 71

Nash, J.C., 52

National Child Benefit (NCB), 156, 163

National child benefit progress report, 2005, The, 165

National Children's Agenda (NCA), 156

National Commission for the Protection of Human Subjects of Biomedical and Behavioral Research, 32–33

National Council of Welfare, 155–57, 161–62, 167

National Institutes of Health (U.S.), 30

National Population Health Survey, 25

Native American postcolonial psychology, 71

Natural Sciences and Engineering Research Council of Canada (NSERC), 27, 32

naturalism: and definition of health, 9, 12–13

Nature of disease, The, 19

Navarro, V., 39, 43, 52

neo-liberalism, 153; as affecting public policy, 164; and globalization, 151, 164; and impacts on health, xxiv, 163. *See also* welfare state

Neuman, M., 166

New Democratic Party (SK), 78–79, 157

New Directions in Population Health Research: Linking Theory, Ethics, and Practice, vii, xi, xii

New public finance: Responding to global challenges, The, 167

Nicolescu, B., xviii, xxv

Nicomachean Ethics, 14, 17

Nielsen, T., 116, 131

Niesen-Vertommen, S., 115–16, 131

Nilson, J., 83

1995 budget and block funding, The, 167

Nisbett, Richard, 59, 63, 72

Norbeck, J.S., 135, 149

Nordenfelt, L., 13, 17, 19

Norenzayan, A., 59, 72

normativism: and definition of health, 9, 12–14

North, F., 51

Nova Scotia Commission on Health Care, 74, 92

Novins, D.K., 20, 33

Nowatzki, Nadine, xxi, xxii

Nulman, I., 136, 149

Nuremberg Code, 27, 32–33

O

Oakley, A., 93, 110

Oaks, Laury, 94, 105–6, 110

O'Connor, T.G., 135, 148–49

OECD *thematic review of early childhood education and care—Canadian background report*, 165

Olivotto, I., 131

On the nature of health: An action-theoretic approach, 19

On the normal and pathological, 32

O'Neil, J.D., 30, 33, 94, 110

Ong, W., 60, 72

Ontario, Government of, 90

Operationalization and research strategy, 32

Orality and literacy: The technologizing of the world, 72

Organization for Economic Cooperation and Development (OECD), ix, 155

Orsini, M., 167

Oths, K.S., xvi, xxv

Ottawa Charter for health promotion, 74, 92

Our children. Our promise. Our future. Early childhood development progress report 2004/2005, 165

Oxford handbook of public policy, The, 165

P

Palmer, J.D., 65, 72

Pamuk, E., 50–51

Paradigm shift: Globalization and the Canadian state, 167

parental leave policy, 161

Park, C., 116, 131

Parker, S., 150

Parra-Medina, D., 43, 46–47, 53

Parry, D., 116, 130–31

Pasarin, M., 52

Patel, D., 51

Payne, D., 127, 131

Pearce, N., 39–40, 47, 52

peer support group, 120

Peng, K., 59, 72

Peoples of the river valleys: The odyssey of the Delaware Indians, 73

Perinatal mental health: A guide to the Edinburgh Postnatal Depression Scale, 148

Personal persistence, identity development, and suicide, 71

Peterson, A.R., 95, 110

Petrucka, P., xxv, 33

Pewewardy, C., 72

Phelan, J., 50

Phillips, C., 130

Philosophical discourse of modernity, The, 72

Physics, 17

Pickett, K.E., 36, 41, 53

Pikhart, H., 47, 52

Pimple, K.D., xxi, 22, 27, 33; ethical questions of, 21, 29, 31–32

Platt, R.W., 110

Plested, B., 33

Polanyi, M., xxv

Polese, M., 163, 167

Polevychok, C., 160, 164

policy making, xiii-xiv; privatization of, 153. *See also* public policy

Politics, 17

Politics of women's health: Exploring agency and autonomy, The, 110

Pong, R., xvi, xxv, 89

Popay, P., 50

population health, vii, ix-x, xii-xiii, 3, 12, 16, 82, 139–40; and child health, xv, 154; definition of health for, 4, 7–11, 13–14, 16; determinants of, viii, xiii, xix, 88; and health promotion, 144, 147; objectives of, 5–6, 12, 15; policies for, 4, 13–14, 16, 134, 153; and prenatal depression, 133–34, 140, 146. *See also* health; health determinants

Population health: Concepts and methods, 168

"Population Health: Defining Health," 6

Population health policy: Federal, provincial and territorial perspectives, 19

Population health policy: Issues and options, 19

population health research, viii, x, xii, xiv, xvii, xix, xxi, xxiv, 22; and Aboriginals, 70; ethical dimensions of, 20–21, 29, 31; framework for, 24, 29, 31; and health definition, 4, 13–14, 16; transdisciplinary nature of, xviii, xx, xxiii

Population Health Template: Key elements and actions that define a population health approach, The, 8, 19

Population Health Template Working Tool, 2005, The, 149

Pörn, I., 19

Porter, R., 18

Portes, A., 39, 46, 52

Postcolonial theory: A critical introduction, 72

Postpartum depression and child development, 148

Potvin, L., 22, 33

Poudrier, J., 111

poverty, viii-x, xvii, xxii, 35, 38–39, 44, 154–54; as cause of depression, 140; and children, ix, 155–57, 163; and health disparities, 15, 36, 43

Poverty and policy in Canada: Implications for health and quality of life, 52, 167

pregnancy: depression during, 133–36, 139, 144, 146–47; medicalization of, 93–95; outcomes of, 94, 141. *See also* depression; fetal health; prenatal care

prenatal care, 133, 135–36, 141. *See also* pregnancy; women

primary health care, 83

Prince Edward Island Ministry of Health, 75, 92

Pringle, B., 160, 167

Privatization, law, and the challenge to feminism, 165

Pro-action, postponement, and preparation/support: A framework for action to reduce the rate of teen pregnancy in Canada, 110

Progressive Conservative Party (Fed), 158

Progressive Conservative Party (SK), 157

Protecting Indigenous knowledge and heritage: A global challenge, 71

Prothrow-Stith, D., 50

Prus, R., 117, 132

Public Health Agency of Canada (PHAC), 4, 6–7, 19, 93–94, 110, 140, 149

Public health and preventative medicine in Canada, 149

public policy. *See* child-relevant public policy; health care policy; housing policy; parental leave policy; social policy

Pushor, D., 167

Putland, C., 53

Putnam, R., 39, 46, 52

Q

Qualitative data analysis, 110

quality of life, vii, 116, 136

Quandt, S.A., 96, 109

Quebec referendum, 153

Quesenberry Jr, C., 119, 132

Quigley, D., 30, 34

Quiroga, A., 52

R

Rabheru, K., 136, 149

Raghunathan, T., 51

Rainbow Report: Our vision for health, The, 90

Ram, R., 37, 52

Raphael, D., 35, 38, 42, 44–45, 48–50, 52, 156, 167

Rapport de la Commission d'Enquete sur les Services de Sante et les Services Sociaux, 92

Rasanen, P., 149

Rasmussen, K., 75, 78, 92

Ratcliffe, P., 45, 52

Ratner, P.A., 19, 90

RBC Community Development Fund, 147

Reading, J.R., 94, 110

Reclaiming Indigenous voice and vision, 71

Redesigning social assistance: Preparing for the new century, 165

Reed, M., xxv

Regan, T., 18

Regina, University of, xi, xviii

Regional Health Authorities (RHAS), 79, 83–85

Regional Health Forum: WHO South-East Asia Region, 150

regionalization: of health boards, 75–76, 86

Regionalization and devolution: Transforming health, reshaping politics?, 91

Regionalization: Where has all the power gone? A Survey of Canadian decision-makers in health care regionalization, 90

Rehnsfeldt, A., 127, 130

Reigle, B., 128, 132

Rein, M., 165

Report of the Commissioner for the Saskatchewan Health Services Survey, 92

Report of the Manitoba Regional Health Authority External Review Committee, 90

Report of the Nova Scotia Commission on Health Care: Towards a new strategy, The, 92

Report of the Royal Commission on Aboriginal Peoples, 71

Report on Plans and Priorities 2007–2008, 19

Report to the Minister of Labour on the minimum wage and other matters under section 15 of the Labour Standards Act, 167

research ethics boards (REB), 27

Research methods in psychology, 130

Responding to The Global Burden of Disease, 148

Restructuring of the Canadian welfare state: Ideology and policy, The, 164

Reznek, Lawrie, 17, 19

Richman, K.A., 5, 13, 17, 19
Riggs, K.W., 149
Rizzini, I., 168
Robertson, A., 90
Robson, K.M., 148
Rochon, J., 74, 77, 92
Rodriguez-Sanz, M., 52
Rogers, R., 77, 92
Romanow, Roy, xvi, xxv, 79, 89
Room, G.J., 44, 52
Rorty, A.O., 60, 72
Rose, N., 96, 111
Rose, R., 52
Rosenberg, M.W., xvi, xxv
Ross, D.P., 109, 111, 166
Ross, N., 50, 52
Royal Commission on Aboriginal Peoples, 64, 71
Royal Commission on the Economic Union and Development Prospects for Canada, 152
Royal University Hospital Foundation (SK), 147
Ruggeri, J., 153, 163, 167
Ruggiero, L., 150
Ruhl, L., 94, 111

S

Sadock, B.J., 148
Sadock, V.A., 148
Saint-Martin, D., 162, 167
Sallot, J., 57, 73
Sancton, A., 163, 167
Sanderson, K., xvii, xxv
Sandman, C.A., 110
Sanmartin, C., 52
Sari, N., xxv
Saskatchewan Child Benefit (SCB), 157, 163
Saskatchewan Education, 159
Saskatchewan Employment Supplement (SES), 157
Saskatchewan, Government of, 156–57, 160, 162–63, 165

Saskatchewan Health, xv, xxv, 75, 77, 82, 92
Saskatchewan Health Research Foundation (SHRF) Nursing Care Partnership, 147
Saskatchewan: Healthy people, a healthy province. Health research strategy, xxv
Saskatchewan Housing Corporation (SHC), 160
Saskatchewan Minimum Wage Board, 161, 167
Saskatchewan politics into the twenty-first century, 89, 167
Saskatchewan Population Health and Evaluation Research Unit (SPHERU), xi-xviii, xx-xxi, 147
Saskatchewan, University of, xi, xviii, 134, 147
Saskatchewan vision for health, A, 92
Saskatchewan vision for health: A framework for change, A, 79, 92
Saskatchewan vision for health: Challenges and opportunities, A, 79, 92
Saskatoon Catholic School Division, 159
Saskatoon, City of, 160, 165
Saskatoon Community Clinic, 149; Westside Clinic of, 136–37, 144, 146–47
Saskatoon Health Region, 136, 147
Saskatoon Housing Authority, 160
Saskatoon Public School Division, 159
Saunders, D., 89
Saunders, R., 161, 167
Scambler, G., 42, 47, 52
Schauffler, E.M., 60, 73
Schei, B., 110
Schnarch, B., 30, 34

Schoenbach, V., 130
School-aged children across Canada: A patchwork of public policies, 166
Schulz, A.J., 46, 52
Schulz, R., 115, 131
Schutt, A.C., 65, 73
Schwarzer, R., 116, 132
Science and Native American communities: Legacies of pain, visions of promise, 72
Scutchfield, F.D., 77, 92
Seaton, P., 74, 77, 92
Segal, M.T., 53
Seguin, L., 110
self-government, rights of: and suicide rates, 68–69
Sen, A., 36, 52
Senate of Canada, 11, 15–16, 19; Subcommittee on Population Health, 16
Sensible guide to a healthy pregnancy, 93, 110
Seto, M., 135, 149
Shah, C.P., 139, 142, 149
Shand, S., 34
Sharp, J., 65, 72
Shaw, M., 51
Shaw, P., 73
Shaw, Rhona, xxiii
Sherwin, S., 110
Shi, L., 38, 43, 51–52
Shibuya, K., 149
Shields, C., 116, 130
Shillington, E.R., 109, 111
Shim, J.K., 94, 96, 111
Siddiqi, A., 154, 166
Side, K., 77, 86, 92
Siedule, T., 161, 166
Sigerist, H., 92
Simard, L., 80
Simpson, J.W., 65, 73
Sinclair, R., xv, xxv, 22, 33
Sitting Bull, 65
Skinner, D., 61, 72
Skogstad, G., 164, 167–68

Sleep, M., 128, 132
Smith, C., 69, 73, 78
Smith, D., 92
Smith, M., 167
Smith, N., 152, 167
Smith, P., 89
Smith, R., xv, xxv
Smye, V., 94, 109
Smylie, J., xvi, xxv
Sobel, R., 5, 19
social assistance, 156–57, 162–63. *See also* social programs; workfare
Social assistance statistical report, 166
social capital, 38–40, 44–45, 47–48
social cohesion, 39–40, 43, 45, 47, 154
Social determinants of health: Canadian perspectives, 50, 52
Social determinants of health: The solid facts, 53
social differences, xxiii, 103, 108; and effects on health, vii-viii, x, 36, 41, 47, 94–95; and expert knowledge, 96, 98–99, 101–2, 105–6. *See also* health disparities; knowledge, expert
Social epidemiology, 50–51
social exclusion, 44–45, 47; framework for, 44
social housing, ix, 154, 160. *See also* social programs
social inequalities. *See* social differences
social investment strategy, 162, 164
Social policies, family types, and child outcomes in selected OECD countries, 166
social policy, 153–55, 161, 163
social programs, ix, 154, 162

Social Sciences and Humanities Research Council of Canada (SSHRC), 27, 32
social status. *See* socioeconomic status
social support: for cancer survivors, 120; as health determinant, 116
Social sustainability of cities: Diversity and the management of change, The, 167
socio-economic status (SES), 38, 40; as health determinant, vii-viii, xiv, 15, 35
Sokol, B., 57, 67–69, 71
Space, gender, knowledge: Feminist readings, 72
Spinelli, M.G., 136, 149
Spirito, A., 135, 150
Spooner, C., 89
Stamp, G.E., 136, 150
Standing Committee on Health Care, 79, 83
Stansfield, D., 51
Starfield, B., 38, 40, 51
Stark, A., 5, 19
Statistics Canada, 32, 109, 164
Staunaes, D., 46, 53
Stein, C., 149
Stephens, C., 45–46, 53
Steps on the road to medicare: Why Saskatchewan led the way, 90
Sternfeld, B., 119, 132
Stevenson, N., xv, xxv
Stewart, N., 148
Stoddart, G., 139, 149, 155, 166
Stren, R., 163, 167
Structural adjustment of capitalism in Saskatchewan, 168
Subramanian, S.V., 37, 49, 53
suicide, xxii, 35, 136. *See also* Aboriginal youth
Suicide, 50
Sullivan, M., 127, 131

Sullivan, T., 74, 90–91
Summary report of flexible child care for flexible workers, 165
Sword, Wendy, 105, 111
Symbolic interaction and ethnographic research. Intersubjectivity and the study of lived human experience, 132
Szreter, S., 47, 53

T

Tait, C., 27, 34
Taking action on population health: A position paper for Health Promotions and Programs Branch staff, 19
Tan, L.K., 109
Tanzi, V., 153, 167
Tataryn, I.V., 94, 111
Taub, D., 123, 130
Taxing illusions: Taxation, democracy and embedded political theory, 90
Taylor, H.A., 21, 28–30, 34, 77, 89
Taylor, J., 92
Taylor, M.G., 92
Taylor, S., 118, 130
Teeple, G., 152, 154, 164, 167
Teucher, Ulrich, xxii, 58, 62, 68, 71–72
Texts, facts, and femininity: Exploring the relations of ruling, 92
Theberge, N., 123, 132
Thomas, C., 50
Thomas, Geraldine, 107, 109
Thomas-MacLean, R., 128, 132
Thompson, L., 30, 34
Thompson, R., 154, 168
Thompson, S., 155, 157, 159, 161, 166
Throwing like a girl and other essays in feminist philosophy and social theory, 132

Tibblin, G., 130

Tilden, V.P., 135, 149

Titus, J.B., 150

Tomijima, N., 149

Torgerson, R., 52, 151, 166

Townsend, P., 35, 53

Transdisciplinarity—Theory and practice, xxv

Transforming New Brunswick's health-care system: The Provincial Health Plan 2008–2012, 92

Transitional Employment Allowance (TEA), 158

Transitional employment allowance, flat rate utilities, rental housing supplements and poverty in Saskatchewan, 166

Trends in income distribution in the post-World War II period: Evidence and interpretation, 165

Tri-council policy statement: Ethical conduct for research involving humans, 27–29, 32

Triandis, H.C., 59, 73

Tritter, J., 77, 87, 92

Turnell, R.W., 109

Turning to earth: Stories of ecological conversion, 73

Tuzzio, L., xxv

21st century employment system for Canada: Guide to the employment insurance legislation, A, 165

2005 annual report, 165

U

Understanding the policy landscape of early childhood development in Saskatchewan, 167

Unemployment Insurance (UI): and restructuring UI/EI system, 160

UNESCO, 32, 34

Unhealthy societies: The afflictions of inequality, 53

Unhealthy times: Political economy perspectives on health and care, 49

Unipolar depression: A lifetime perspective, 149

Universal Declaration of Bioethics and Human Rights, 27, 32

Unruh, A., 115–16, 132

V

Vaillancourt, F., 156, 158, 166

Valaskakis, G., 34, 71

Valonen, P., 149

Van De Veer, D., 18

van Doorslaer, E., 37, 53

Veenstra, G., 43, 45, 53, 75, 77, 86, 91–92

Veijola, J., 149

Verges, N., 52

Volpe, A.G., 150

W

Wade, R.H., 154, 168

Wadhwa, P.D., 110

Wagner, E., 130

Wagstaff, A., 37, 53

Waldfogel, J., 166

Waller, G., 135, 148

Wallerstein, N., 154, 168

Wallwork, E., 28–29, 34

Wanke, M., 89

Ward, G.K., 69, 73

Warnock, J.W., 159, 168

Waterproof 2: Canada's drinking water report card, 18

Waters, A., 59, 66, 71, 73

Weber, L., 43, 46–47, 53

Weed, D.L., 22, 34

Welfare incomes, 2006–2007, 167

welfare state, ix-x, 43, 74, 78; retrenchment of, 152–53, 161–62. *See also* social programs

Wenman, W.M., 94, 111

Wennemo, I., 36, 53

Wermuth, L., 35, 42, 53

Western knowledge systems, 70

Wetherell, M., 77, 90

Wetzel, K., 74, 76, 78, 92

Wharf Higgins, J., 86, 90, 92

What is disease?, 18

What works? A first look at evaluating Manitoba's regional health programs and policies at the population level, 33

Whitaker, R.C., 135, 149

White, L.A., 158–59, 168

Whittle, K.L., 46–47, 53

Wiegers, W., 162–63, 168

Wield-Anderson, L., 148

Wilkerson, D.S., 135, 150

Wilkins, R., 110

Wilkinson, D., 77, 92

Wilkinson, R.G., 36, 38–39, 41, 44, 47, 51, 53, 154, 168

Williams, A.S., xxv, 22, 95, 116, 136, 150

Williams, G.H., 34

Williams, J.I., 91

Williams, R., 131

Williams, S.J., 111

Wilmoth, M., 125, 132

Wilson, K., xvi, xxv

Wing, S., 30, 34

Wodak, R., 77, 92

Wolfson, M., 50, 52

women: and depression, 134, 145–46; maternal agency of, 94–95, 99–100, 102–3; mental health of, 140. *See also* depression; pregnancy

Woods, J., 75, 86, 91

Woods, X., 125, 130

Woolcock, M., 47, 53

workfare, 157–58, 162–63

World Health Organization
(WHO), 19, 21, 77, 80,
92, 134, 139, 150; and
health definition,
4–7
World Medical Association,
32, 34
World risk society, 109
World Summit for
Children, 155
Wormald, H., 128, 132
Wulu, J., 51

X

Xu, H., 149

Y

Yadlon, S., 125, 132
*Yearning for the land: A
search for the importance
of place,* 73
Yen, I., 51
Yip, A.S.K., 148
Yngwe, M.A., 42, 53
Young, I.M., 125, 132
Young, K., 123, 132
Young, T.K., 154, 168
Youngblood Henderson, J.,
59, 62–64, 66, 71

Z

Ziersch, a.m., 45, 53
Zola, I., 93, 111
Zuckerman, B.S., 135, 150

The body of this book is set in *Arno*. Named after the river that runs through Florence, the center of the Italian Renaissance, *Arno* draws on the warmth and readability of early humanist types of the 15th and 16th centuries. While inspired by the past, *Arno* is distinctly contemporary in both appearance and function. Designed by Robert Slimbach, Adobe principal designer, *Arno* is a meticulously crafted face in the tradition of early Venetian and Aldine book types. Embodying themes that Slimbach has explored in typefaces such as *Minion*® and *Brioso*™, *Arno* represents a distillation of his design ideals and a refinement of his craft.

The accents in this book are set in *Rockwell*, a distinctive version of a geometric slab serif design, which has retained its popularity since its appearance in the 1930s. The slab serifs, or Egyptians, originated in the nineteenth century when they were used principally for display work. The first of the *Rockwell* fonts was issued by Monotype in 1934. It is a prime example of this twentieth century approach. The sturdy design of *Rockwell* is given a particular sparkle by angular terminals.